MARTIN J. CLINE, M.D.

Associate Director, Cancer Research Institute, and Associate Professor of Medicine,
School of Medicine, University of California, San Francisco

CANCER
CHEMOTHERAPY

VOLUME

I

IN THE SERIES

MAJOR PROBLEMS IN INTERNAL MEDICINE

Lloyd H. Smith, Jr., M.D., *Editor*

W. B. SAUNDERS COMPANY · PHILADELPHIA · LONDON · TORONTO

W. B. Saunders Company: West Washington Square
                          Philadelphia, Pa.   19105

                          12 Dyott Street
                          London, WC1A   1DB

                          1835 Yonge Street
                          Toronto 7, Ontario

616.994
C64c
v. 1

Cancer Chemotherapy — M.I.P.M. — *Vol. I*   ISBN   0-7216-2605-X

Library of Congress catalog card number 72-135320.

Print No.:   9   8   7   6   5   4   3

FOREWORD

This book represents the first of a new series of monographs which will appear under the title "Major Problems in Internal Medicine." In a time of a population explosion of books even greater than that of men, announcements of new publications may not be cause for elation. It has been gently suggested that one should not speak unless he can improve on silence. Has this wise restraint been honored in these projected publications? Only time will tell, but their genesis is as follows.

The physician has a finite number of receptor mechanisms against which beat a plethora of periodicals named for disciplines or diseases, organ systems or secretions. The result may be competitive inhibition. Virtually any article submitted, whatever its merit or lack thereof, eventually finds publication as it filters down the cascade of journalistic acceptability. The majority at best represent microadvances in continuing problems; at worst they misinform or merely rearrange our ambiguities. Yet clearly we live in an exciting time for medical research and medical care. The new sophistications of biology are being increasingly transcribed and translated into tangible gains by elucidating human physiology in health and disease. In the first half of this century physics stood at the apex of science. In the second half molecular biology holds this position and medicine is the conduit through which its achievements flow most readily into practical application. Many scientists, physicians and physician-scientists participate in this continuum of research activity. All physicians and their patients are the beneficiaries of the new medical science which has resulted and which will continue to evolve in our time.

The problem remains—how can these advances in medicine be most effectively summarized in a form of greatest usefulness to the profession? The specialty article is of necessity narrow in scope, usually free-floating rather than properly set in the overall field. The textbook because of its encyclopedic dimensions must usually compress a single subject into terse but colorless epigrams. Between these two extremes the analytical review emerges with increasing importance as the best method for bringing form and coherence to science.

Such reviews must judge, not merely recite. They must bear the intellectual imprint of the author, not the codified print-out of the computer. The monographs in "Major Problems in Internal Medicine" will attempt to provide this type of selective summary and analysis for topics in medicine on a continuing basis. The books will appear when three conditions have been met: (a) a topic is chosen as one of importance for the physician; (b) recent advances or changing concepts call for reevaluation of that topic; (c) an author is available who can write about it with authority, judgment and clarity. Because of these conditions the monographs will not appear in a systematic sequence, as sections of a textbook would be arranged. Their publication will be opportunistic. The reader's attention is directed to the titles in preparation for this series, a list of which appears opposite the title page. The time of publication of the various monographs cannot be precisely predicted, but each promises to be an important study of a specific area in internal medicine by a writer or writers who have contributed to its elucidation.

The medical treatment of malignant disease is often complex, frustrating and charged with eventual failure. So is that of congestive heart failure, but the latter condition does not usually convey the same sense of hopelessness in patient and physician alike. In fact, one could say, so is life itself although it is rarely rejected out of hand. By slow accretion of knowledge over several decades, the treatment of malignant diseases has made substantial advances. As a result the physician often is able to reduce disability and prolong life. Sometimes he is able to cure. At the present time the modalities of therapy are largely toxic or injurious to all cells, and selectivity of response depends on comparative vulnerability of normal and abnormal cells. Such agents are useful and still the most frequently used, as reviewed in this book. It is clear that this approach must be and will be supplanted in the future by more specific mechanisms, whether they are metabolic (such as antifolics in choriocarcinoma or asparaginase in leukemia), immunologic or antimicrobial.

In this monograph, Dr. Martin Cline, who is the Associate Director of the Cancer Research Institute at the University of California San Francisco Medical Center, has written a scholarly review of the medical treatment of malignant diseases. He has managed to summarize in a very lucid fashion the scientific basis of therapy as well as the practicalities of clinical application in this complex and rapidly changing field. *Cancer Chemotherapy* should be a useful source book for all physicians who treat patients with malignant diseases.

LLOYD H. SMITH, JR.

PREFACE

Cancer chemotherapy is just emerging from its infancy and achieving identity as a distinct clinical discipline. Consistent successful use of cytotoxic agents was unknown before 1945, and the number of useful agents was extremely limited before 1950. Since then, the field has been in an exponential growth phase. Traditionally the management of the patient with malignant disease has been in the hands of the surgeon and the radiation therapist. With the advent of new drugs and the growth of knowledge of the pharmacodynamics of chemotherapeutic agents and of cellular proliferation, the chemotherapist has become an essential figure on the team of physicians required to treat properly the patient with malignant disease.

Formerly a chemotherapist was usually a clinical investigator trying to establish the conditions under which a given agent was useful in treating a given neoplastic disease. Recently, however, a new group has been emerging. The modern chemotherapist functions primarily as a practitioner. He is usually a physician with a background in internal medicine or hematology and with a special interest in oncology and clinical pharmacology, responding to the challenge of malignant disease and the increasing number and complexity of chemotherapeutic agents.

The chemotherapist may be any well-trained physician with an interest in malignant disease who is willing to observe a few guidelines. He must always ask himself: What are the indications for treatment of a given malignant disease? What beneficial result for the patient can be expected from drug therapy? What are the possible harmful side effects of a given drug, and what are the warning signs of its toxicity?

It is my objective in this volume to summarize the available information in the rapidly changing field of cancer chemotherapy for the postgraduate student, the house officer, and the practicing physician.

MARTIN J. CLINE

Acknowledgments

I am indebted to Ruth M. Hassler for her patient, thoughtful, and perceptive editing of the manuscript; to Gwen Dangerfield for her extraordinarily patient and precise secretarial assistance; and to Doctors Alfred de Lorimier, Howard F. Morrelli, and Sydney E. Salmon for their careful reviews of parts of the manuscript.

CONTENTS

CHAPTER 1

INTRODUCTION TO CHEMOTHERAPY

The modern era of chemotherapy was ushered in by the introduction of the polyfunctional alkylating agents in the early 1940's. By
1950 the rate of introduction of useful new agents had begun to
accelerate; folic acid antagonists, purine analogues, and adrenocorticosteroids appeared in rapid succession. By 1960 whole new classes
of antitumor agents had become available. The principal historical
developments in cancer chemotherapy are summarized briefly in
Table 1–1.[1-19]

It is apparent that the field of chemotherapy is new and that
its growth has been rapid. Its complexities seem to be rivaled only by
those of blood coagulation. Fortunately, however, there are certain
unifying concepts that aid in the selection and rational use of chemotherapeutic agents.

MODE OF ACTION OF CANCER CHEMOTHERAPEUTIC AGENTS

DNA Synthesis and the Cell Replication Cycle

Malignant tissues are made up largely of dividing cells that
synthesize DNA at some point in their life cycle. Most useful chemotherapeutic agents have as their principal mode of action either
interruption of DNA synthesis or combination with DNA macromole-
cules (Fig. 1–1). An undesirable consequence of this drug action is

1

TABLE 1-1   Development of Chemotherapeutic Agents

Approximate Date	References (Numbers)	Agent	Diseases Treated
1865	1	Potassium arsenite	Leukemias, various malignancies
1893	2	Coley's toxins	Various malignancies
1941–1945	3	Estrogens	Carcinoma of prostate and breast
	4	Androgens	Advanced carcinoma of breast
	5, 6	Nitrogen mustard	Lymphomas, solid tumors
1948–1950	7	Adrenocorticosteroids	Leukemias, lymphomas, multiple myeloma
	8	6-Mercaptopurine	Acute leukemia
	9	Antifolates	Acute leukemia, choriocarcinoma
	10	Busulfan	Chronic myelocytic leukemia
1955	11, 12	Actinomycin-D	Wilms' tumor, testicular tumors, choriocarcinoma, neuroblastoma
	13	5-Fluorouracil	Carcinoma of gastrointestinal tract, advanced carcinoma of breast
1960–1964	14	Progestins	Endometrial carcinoma
	15	Vinca alkaloids	Lymphomas, reticuloendothelial malignancies of childhood, acute lymphoblastic leukemia, choriocarcinoma
	16	Cytosine arabinoside	Acute leukemia, disseminated lymphomas
	17	o, p'-DDD	Adrenal carcinoma
1964–1968	18	Daunomycin	Acute leukemia, neuroblastoma
	19	L-Asparaginase	Acute lymphoblastic leukemia

that those normal tissues that have a high rate of cellular proliferation bear the brunt of toxic side effects. These tissues are the normal bone marrow elements, the gastrointestinal epithelial cells, and the cells of the hair follicles and skin. Evidence of toxicity is seen clinically as follows:

Bone marrow: anemia, leukopenia (infection), thrombocytopenia (bleeding)
Gastrointestinal tract: diarrhea, vomiting, nausea, surface ulcerations
Hair follicles: alopecia

The second concept important to the use of anticancer drugs is that not all agents are equally effective throughout the cellular life cycle.[20] Obviously drugs interfering with DNA synthesis are active

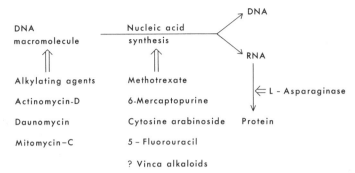

Figure 1-1 Site of action of chemotherapeutic agents.

against proliferating cells as opposed to resting cells, and are most effective during that period in the cell cycle in which DNA is actively being synthesized. Such drugs are active against tumors with a high rate of cellular proliferation, as, for example, in acute leukemia. These drugs are relatively ineffective against tumors with a slow rate of proliferation, only a small fraction of whose cells are synthesizing DNA at any given time. Examples of such slowly growing tumors are chronic lymphocytic leukemia and many solid tumors. For such slowly growing tumors, agents active against resting cells as well as cells actively synthesizing DNA are necessary. Nitrogen mustard and chlorambucil are examples of drugs active against some slowly growing tumors.

CELL CYCLE. The concept of drug activity during only a phase of the life cycle of proliferating malignant cells is becoming of increasing importance to both the theoretical and the practical aspects of cancer therapy.[20] It is worth reviewing this cycle (Fig. 1-2). A convenient place to start in the life cycle of the cell is with the initiation of division (mitosis). Mitosis occupies a discrete phase of the life cycle, which is designated D for division. After the cell has

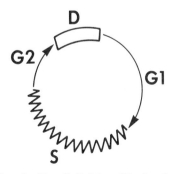

Figure 1-2 The cell cycle: D, cell division; G1, the phase preceding active DNA synthesis; S, the phase of DNA synthesis; G2, the premitotic resting phase.

completed its division, it enters the G1 phase, which for a long time was considered by cell biologists to be relatively quiescent. Emerging from G1, the cell begins a phase of active DNA synthesis, which has been termed the S phase. After completion of DNA synthesis, the cell again enters a resting phase before initiation of mitosis; this phase of apparent rest is called G2.

Certain interesting features of this cycle have emerged during the past few years. Traditionally, morphologists had concentrated on the rather dramatic events of mitosis and cell division with its formation of the spindle, separation of the chromosomes, and related events. It is only recently that other aspects of the cycle have received attention. Certain features of the cycle are now evident. In most dividing cells the periods for DNA synthesis (S), the G2 phase, and division (D) are relatively fixed in time and of nearly constant duration. Variation of the length of the cell cycle generally occurs in the G1 phase. When cells stop proliferating and come to rest, they do so in the G1 phase, not in the S, G2, or division phases. For example, after partial hepatectomy and subsequent hepatic proliferation, the liver cells stop dividing and are arrested in the G1 phase.

The G1 phase is not at all the inactive period it was once thought to be. Active RNA synthesis and protein synthesis occur during this interval. The duration of this phase seems to be related in some way to the proliferative activity of the tissues: When proliferative activity is high, the G1 phase is short; when proliferative activity is low, the G1 phase tends to be long. In very rapidly proliferating protozoa, in the early embryo, and in certain malignant tissues, the G1 phase may be so short as to be essentially obscured.

It is not clear, at present, how a differentiated mammalian cell receives instruction to leave the G1 phase and begin DNA synthesis. Most of our information in this subject comes from the study of microorganisms.[21, 22] There is evidence in higher life forms that the control mechanism requires interaction between the nucleus and cytoplasm of the replicating cell. Once the S phase begins, several things happen in rapid succession. The enzymes necessary for DNA synthesis, including those of purine and pyrimidine biosynthesis, and those necessary for formation of macromolecular nucleic acids increase in specific activity. After the DNA content of the cell has doubled, the phase of DNA synthesis is complete and the cell enters the G2 phase. This phase was once thought to be a quiescent period, but it is now quite clear that RNA synthesis and protein synthesis are required before the cell can construct a mitotic apparatus and begin division.

These considerations are critical to the action of chemotherapeutic agents. As a generalization, it can be said that replicating cells are sensitive to attack by the commonly used antimetabolites only during the S phase. It is probable that the G2 phase is the point of the cellular life cycle at which certain mitotic inhibitors exert their effect.

Agents that are effective mainly during a particular phase of the cell cycle, for example, cellular DNA synthesis, are called *cell cycle-specific*. Those whose action is prolonged and independent of DNA synthesis are called *cell cycle-nonspecific*. This distinction between specific and nonspecific agents is relative rather than absolute. It is obvious, however, that the agents that are most effective during the S phase will be relatively ineffective in slowly turning over cell populations with a high percentage of dormant cells. On the other hand, alkylating agents and other drugs interacting primarily with macromolecular DNA (e.g., actinomycin-D) seem to be largely independent of the stage of the cell replication cycle and are often effective against tumors with relatively low proliferative activity.

AVAILABLE AGENTS

The number of classes of clinically useful chemotherapeutic agents is limited at present. By familiarizing himself with the types of useful drugs, the chemotherapist greatly simplifies the choice of drug. The classes of chemotherapeutic compounds, examples of each class, the cell cycle specificity, and the general usefulness of these compounds are summarized in Table 1–2.

Armed with this impressive list of potent and potentially harmful drugs, and faced with the patient who has an advanced or inoperable malignancy, the chemotherapist must always ask himself: What are the indications for treatment? These indications involve a general knowledge of the natural history or behavior of the malignancy and specific knowledge of the extent of disease, rapidity of advance, and previous treatment in the individual patient.

Guidelines for Use

It is critically important to establish and to observe certain basic tenets in using any of the cancer chemotherapeutic agents in a clinical setting. The wise physician observes the following tenets each time he treats a patient with malignant disease:

1. Use chemotherapeutic agents only when a diagnosis of malignancy has been established histologically.

2. Follow several parameters that will objectively reflect the response of the tumor to the chemotherapeutic agent.

3. Do not use chemotherapeutic agents unless there are adequate facilities to monitor the potential toxicity of the agent to the patient's normal tissues.

These points are worth elaborating. The difficulties of treating a

TABLE 1-2   *Classes of Chemotherapeutic Agents*

CLASS OF COMPOUND	EXAMPLES	CELL CYCLE SPECIFICITY	DISEASES IN WHICH USEFUL
Alkylating agents	Nitrogen mustard, chlorambucil, cyclo-phosphamide, busulfan	Nonspecific	Lymphomas; many solid tumors; chronic lymphocytic leukemia
Antimetabolites	1. Methotrexate 2. 6-Mercaptopurine 3. Cytosine arabinoside 4. 5-Fluorouracil	Specific	1-3. Acute leukemias 1. Choriocarcinoma 4. Carcinoma of breast; carcinoma of G. I. tract
Antibiotics	1. Actinomycin-D 2. Mithramycin° 3. Daunomycin°	Nonspecific	1. Neuroblastoma; choriocarcinoma 2. Testicular tumors 3. Acute leukemia
Plant alkaloids	1. Vincristine 2. Vinblastine	Specific	1. Acute leukemias; lymphomas 2. Reticuloendothelial malignancy; lym-phomas
Adrenocorticosteroids	Prednisone	? Nonspecific	Lymphocytic leukemias; lymphomas; carci-noma of breast
Other steroids	Estrogens Androgens Progestins	Unknown	Carcinoma of prostate Carcinoma of breast Carcinoma of endo-metrium
Enzymes	L-Asparaginase	Unknown	Acute leukemias; lymphomas

°Clinical use not definitely established.

patient "blindly," without a tissue diagnosis, may be so horrendous that one experience is enough to drive home the lesson that anticancer drugs are never given without a histopathologic diagnosis of malignancy. The commonest situation in which I have seen "blind therapeutic trials" is that of the patient suspected of having lymphoma because of fever, weight loss, constitutional symptoms, and a downhill course. When such patients are subsequently proved to have tuberculosis, occult fungal infections, or carcinoma such as hypernephroma, the prior use of alkylating agents is often an embarrassment to the physician and a disservice to the patient. An extension of this basic tenet of chemotherapy is that these agents are rarely, if ever, used in a diagnostic trial to determine the extent or type of malignancy.

Because chemotherapeutic agents are potentially toxic, it is unreasonable to give them unless one can objectively determine that they are helping the patient. Objective determinations may include, for example, measurement of the patient's performance status, a decrease in the size of the tumor, disappearance of hypercalcemia, disappearance of paraprotein in the serum, or return of an infiltrated marrow to normal. Subjective improvement, such as a decrease in pain, is a less satisfactory indication of drug action, since placebos may have the same effect. Obviously, the potent chemotherapeutic agents should never be used as placebos.

Because of their narrow margin of safety, chemotherapeutic agents should not be used unless the physician is prepared to monitor potential toxicity to normal tissues. This means close and frequent follow-up visits, including history-taking for symptoms of toxicity (e.g., nausea, vomiting, dysuria), a physical examination with particular attention to skin and mucous membranes, a white blood count, and a platelet count. A good look at a blood smear can often substitute for a platelet count in the hands of an experienced observer. With most drugs, the red cell count and hematocrit tend to fall more slowly than the levels of the rapidly turning over leukocytes and platelets; therefore, a stable hematocrit is not an assurance of a lack of toxic side effects. The more important parameters to be followed in patients receiving anticancer drugs are listed in Table 1–3.

CRITERIA FOR EXPERIMENTAL TRIALS. The experimental use of chemotherapeutic agents falls within the province of the clinical investigator. Basic requirements for experimental trials are that useful information be obtained either for the treated patient or for other patients with similar disease and that, insofar as possible, no harmful effects result from the experimental approach. Experimental administration of new or old drugs is not to be undertaken casually. Experimental drugs applied to a single patient almost never yield useful

TABLE 1–3 *Parameters for Tumor Response and Toxicity*

TUMOR RESPONSE

Tumor size: palpation, radiologic measurement, radioisotope scans
Serum calcium: Carcinoma involving bone, myeloma, certain lymphomas
Serum and urinary paraproteins: myeloma, macroglobulinemia
Peripheral white blood count: Leukemia, certain lymphomas
Gonadotropin titer: Choriocarcinoma, certain testicular tumors
Disappearance of effusions: Tumors involving pleural or peritoneal surfaces, or obstructing lymphatics

TOXICITY TO NORMAL TISSUES

Fall in level of normal leukocytes (granulocytes generally tend to fall before lymphocytes)
Fall in platelet level
Fall in hematocrit (often a late finding)
Gastrointestinal symptoms, mucous membrane lesions
Alopecia
Serum uric acid
Special problems with individual drugs (e.g., see Chap. 2, cyclophosphamide, busulfan, vincristine)

information and often do harm. Therefore, new drugs and procedures are usually restricted to medical centers where large numbers of patients are seen and where experimental procedures are rigidly controlled. In this book we are concerned principally with established criteria for drug use, and experimental therapy is cited only when it provides insight into treatment of malignant disease or when such therapy holds great promise for the future.

CRITERIA FOR ESTABLISHED CHEMOTHERAPY. The criteria for the clinical use of a given agent are (1) that the malignancy is known to respond to the agent in a large percentage of cases in a manner beneficial to the patient, or (2) that the drug is a useful adjuvant to either surgery or radiation therapy in the management or cure of malignancy. Like most things in medicine, established criteria for drug use are relative. Some malignancies respond favorably to drugs in virtually all patients treated. Other types of malignant disease will respond only a small fraction of the time. The indications for treatment in the latter situation are influenced by many variables, including extent of disease, rapidity of advance, and social and financial factors.

TABLE 1-4 *Current Status of Clinical Cancer Chemotherapy*

DISEASE	AGENT	BENEFIT
Malignant Diseases Usually Benefited		
Acute lymphoblastic leukemia	Adrenocorticosteroids, vincristine, 6-mercaptopurine, methotrexate, cyclophosphamide	Initial remission > 80%; prolonged survival
Chronic leukemia: Myelocytic	Busulfan, 6-mercaptopurine	Clinical improvement in >70%; occasional prolonged survival
Lymphocytic	Alkylating agents, adrenocorticosteroids	Clinical improvement; occasional prolonged survival
Hodgkin's disease	Alkylating agents, vinca alkaloids, procarbazine	Clinical improvement in >60%
Carcinoma of breast	Estrogens, androgens, 5-fluorouracil, alkylating agents	25–50% response; prolonged survival
Carcinoma of prostate	Estrogens	>80% response; prolonged survival
Trophoblastic tumors	Actinomycin-D, methotrexate, vinca alkaloids, alkylating agents	>80% response, with permanent regression in 70%
Tumors of children: Wilms' tumor	Actinomycin-D, alkylating agents, vincristine	>50% response; prolonged survival
Neuroblastoma	Alkylating agents, actinomycin-D, vincristine	Temporary response, 50%; occasional prolonged response

TABLE 1-4 *Current Status of Clinical Cancer Chemotherapy (Continued)*

DISEASE	AGENT	BENEFIT
Malignant Diseases Often Benefited		
Acute myelocytic leukemia	6-Mercaptopurine, vincristine, cytosine arabinoside	Clinical improvement in 10–30%
Lymphosarcoma	Alkylating agents, adrenocorticosteroids; vinca alkaloids	Occasional clinical improvement and prolonged survival
Reticulum cell sarcoma	Alkylating agents, vinca alkaloids, adrenocorticosteroids	Occasional clinical improvement
Multiple myeloma	Alkylating agents; adrenocorticosteroids	Objective response in 30%; prolonged survival
Carcinoma of bowel and stomach	5-Fluorouracil	Clinical improvement in 15–25%
Carcinoma of ovary	Alkylating agents	Clinical improvement in 30–50%
Carcinoma of endometrium	Progestins	Clinical improvement in 25%
Testicular carcinoma, germinal cell	Actinomycin-D, vincristine, methotrexate, chlorambucil	Clinical improvement in approximately 30%
Adrenal carcinoma	o, p'-DDD	Occasional clinical improvement, sometimes prolonged
Minimal Benefit		
Hepatic, pancreatic tumors	5-Fluorouracil	10% objective response
Melanoma	Alkylating agents, vinca alkaloids	5% objective response
Differentiated sarcoma	Actinomycin-D, cyclophosphamide	5% objective response
Tumors of uterine cervix	Alkylating agents	5% objective response

Table 1–4 lists the types of malignancy in which the patient is usually, often, or seldom benefited by the various drugs, and the frequency of remission usually obtained. This list must be considered as only a general guide. In addition to the diseases listed, there are two other clinical situations in which well-established criteria for chemotherapy exist: recurrent effusions (especially pleural effusions) and meningeal leukemia. In these situations drug treatment is usually local and often very effective.

A number of malignant tumors respond only rarely to chemotherapy. These include carcinomas of the lung, thyroid, kidney, liver, pancreas, and uterine cervix; sarcomas of bone and soft tissues; and melanoma. The decision to treat patients with these malignancies must be made with the realization that the chances of beneficial results are small, that improvement is usually temporary, and that the drugs employed are potentially harmful.

At the present time there are only a few malignancies that can be said to be "cured" by chemotherapy alone. Solid evidence for drug-induced cure exists only for choriocarcinoma and a rare type of lymphoma known as Burkitt's lymphoma. In both, there are probably active immunologic defenses present in the host against antigenically distinct tumor tissues. Similar antigenic differences between normal and malignant tissues probably exist for other tumors, but these differences are probably not as striking either qualitatively or quantitatively as in the case of choriocarcinoma and Burkitt's lymphoma.

PROBLEMS FOR THE FUTURE

Will we ever be able to cure other malignancies by drug therapy? The answer to this question is still unknown, but there is reason for hope. The greatest concerted effort to achieve such an objective has been made in childhood leukemia, a disease involving rapid proliferation of a high proportion of the malignant cells. The achievements in the treatment of this disease have been impressive. Before the early 1950's, the life expectancy of patients with acute lymphoblastic leukemia was usually less than 20 weeks. With the advent of methotrexate and 6-mercaptopurine therapy, this figure rose to approximately 12 months. Now the life expectancy is approaching 18 to 24 months, and many large institutions have a few patients who have survived, two, three, or occasionally four years.

Briefly, the major problems to be solved before further advances can be made are the following. We must learn more about the cycle of replicating malignant cells and attempt to time our therapy with drugs to correspond to that time in the cycle when they are most effective. We must have better means of detecting malignant cells when they are too few in number to produce clinical manifestations. We must learn to identify and manipulate host defense mechanisms, when possible, to combat the malignant process. We must learn more about the pharmacodynamics of chemotherapeutic agents and more about their optimal use clinically. Supportive therapy, including platelet and white cell transfusions, must be made available at lower cost and on a larger scale. When these goals are achieved, perhaps we shall be able to add a number of additional malignant diseases to the list of those curable by drug therapy.

REFERENCES

1. Lissauer in Bendorf, Zwei Fälle von Leucaemie. Berl. Klin. Wschr. Vol. 2, No. 40, 403–404, October 2, 1865.
2. Coley, W. B.: The treatment of malignant tumors by repeated inoculations of erysipelas: with a report of ten original cases. Amer. J. Med. Sci., 105:487–501, 1893.
3. Herbst, W. P.: Effects of estradiol dipropionate and diethyl stilbestrol on malignant prostatic tissue. Trans. Amer. Assoc. Genito-Urin. Surg., 34:195–202, 1941.
4. Loeser, A. A.: Mammary carcinoma. Response to implantation of male hormone and progesterone. Lancet, 2:698–700, 1941.

5. Gilman, A.: The initial clinical trial of nitrogen mustard. Amer. J. Surg., 105:574–578, 1963.
6. Rhoads, C. P.: Nitrogen mustards in the treatment of neoplastic disease. Official statement. J.A.M.A., 131:656–658, 1946.
7. Pearson, O. H., Eliel, L. P., Rawson, R. W., Dobriner, K., and Rhoads, C. P.: ACTH- and cortisone-induced regression of lymphoid tumors in man: A preliminary report. Cancer, 2:943–945, 1949.
8. Burchenal, J. H., Murphy, M. L., Ellison, R. R., Sykes, M. P., Tan, C. T., Leone, L. A., Karnofsky, D. A., Craver, L. F., Dargeon, H. W., and Rhoads, C. P.: Clinical evaluation of a new antimetabolite, 6-mercaptopurine, in the treatment of leukemia and allied diseases. Blood, 8:965, 1953.
9. Farber, S., Diamond, L. K., Mercer, R. D., Sylvester, R. F., Jr., and Wolff, J. A.: Temporary remissions in acute leukemia in children produced by folic acid antagonist, 4-aminopteroylglutamic acid (aminopterin). New Eng. J. Med., 238:787, 1948.
10. Haddow, A., and Timmis, G. M.: Myleran in chronic myeloid leukaemia. Chemical constitution and biological action. Lancet, 1:207–208, 1953.
11. Schulte, G.: Erfahrungen mit neuen cytostatischen Mitteln bei Hämoblastosen und Carcinomen und die Abgrenzung ihrer Wirkungen gegen Röntgentherapie. Z. Krebsforsch., 58:500–503, 1952.
12. Waksman, S. A. (Ed.): The actinomycins and their importance in the treatment of tumors in animals and man. Ann. New York Acad. Sci., 89:283, 1960.
13. Heidelberger, C., and Ansfield, F. J.: Clinical and experimental use of fluorinated pyrimidines in cancer chemotherapy. Cancer Res., 23:1226–1243, 1963.
14. Kelley, R. M., and Baker, W. H.: Progestational agents in the treatment of carcinoma of the endometrium. New Eng. J. Med., 264:216–222, 1961.
15. Johnson, I. S., Armstrong, J. G., Gorman, M., and Burnett, J. P., Jr.: The vinca alkaloids: A new class of oncolytic agents. Cancer Res., 23:1390, 1963.
16. Evans, J. S., Musser, E. A., Mengel, G. D., Forsblad, K. R., and Hunter, J. H.: Antitumor activity of 1-β-D-arabinofuranosylcytosine hydrochloride. Proc. Soc. Exp. Biol. Med., 106:350, 1961.
17. Bergenstal, D. M., Hertz, R., Lipsett, M. B., and Moy, R. H.: Chemotherapy of adrenocortical cancer with o,p'DDD. Ann. Intern. Med., 53:672–682, 1960.
18. Di Marco, A., Gaetani, M., Dorigotti, L., Soldati, M., and Bellini, O.: Experimental studies on the antitumor activity of daunomycin: A new antibiotic with antitumor activity. Tumori, 49:203–217, 1963.
19. Broome, J. D.: Studies on the mechanism of tumor inhibition by L-asparaginase. J. Exp. Med., 127:1055–1072, 1968.
20. Skipper, H. E.: Biochemical, biological, pharmacologic, toxicologic, kinetic and clinical (subhuman and human) relationships. Cancer, 21:600–610, 1968.
21. Pardee, A. B.: Control of cell division: Models from microorganisms. Cancer Res., 28:1802–1809, 1968.
22. Lark, K. G.: Regulation of chromosome replication and segregation in bacteria. Bacteriol. Rev., 30:3–32, 1966.

Additional Recent Bibliography Not Cited in Text

23. Boesen, E., and Davis, W.: Cytotoxic Drugs in the Treatment of Cancer. London, Edward Arnold (Publishers) Ltd. 1969.
24. Feinstein, A. R.: A clinical method for estimating the rate of growth of a cancer. Yale J. Biol. Med., 41:422–433, 1969.
25. Goldin, A.: Factors pertaining to complete drug-induced remission of tumor in animals and man. Cancer Res., 29:2285–2291, 1969.
26. Sartorelli, A. C.: Some approaches to the therapeutic exploitation of metabolic sites of vulnerability of neoplastic cells. Cancer Res., 29:2292–2299, 1969.
27. LePage, G. A., and Kaneko, T.: Effective means of reducing toxicity without concomitant sacrifice of efficacy of carcinostatic therapy. Cancer Res., 29:2314–2318, 1969.
28. Mueller, G. C.: The $G_1 \rightarrow S$ conversion: A target for cancer chemotherapy. Cancer Res., 29:2394–2397, 1964.
29. Handschumacher, R. E.: Structural and regulatory aspects of enzymes in chemotherapy. Cancer Res., 29:2466–2468, 1969.

CHAPTER 2

PHARMACOLOGIC BASIS OF CANCER CHEMOTHERAPY

The purpose of this chapter is to provide an introduction to the pharmacologic basis of chemotherapeutic agents and, in some instances, to analyze the mechanism of action and metabolism of useful drugs. No attempt has been made to be encyclopedic in the pharmacologic characterization of these agents, since this is a book primarily concerned with their clinical use. Whenever possible, the reader has been provided with references to the literature, both original reports and comprehensive review articles.

FACTORS AFFECTING THE USEFULNESS OF DRUGS

Selective Toxicity

The term selective toxicity suggests that the useful chemotherapeutic agents have a greater cytotoxic effect on malignant tissues than on the normal cells of the tumor-bearing host. If the differences between the malignant and normal cells were qualitative, the problem of selective toxicity would be relatively simple. Unfortunately the differences between normal and neoplastic seem to be largely quantitative. Nevertheless, these quantitative differences can also be exploited usefully in chemotherapy. Such differences relate to the levels of activity of certain enzymes, the rates of cellular aerobic and anaerobic metabolism, and the rates of cellular proliferation and associated macromolecular synthesis, including DNA, RNA, and protein synthesis.

Many cancer cells have a high rate of proliferation; consequently, they are susceptible to interference with their supply and utilization

12

of critical building blocks, such as amino acids, purines, pyrimidines, and one-carbon components. Such cancer cells also require intact macromolecular DNA for replication and are damaged by cytotoxic agents that disrupt nuclear materials or change the configuration of nucleic acids. These characteristics of malignant tissue might suffice for the development of a completely successful system of chemotherapy were it not for the fact that certain normal tissues also have a high proliferative capacity rivaling and in some instances exceeding that of malignant tissues. Such normal tissues, including bone marrow elements, gastrointestinal epithelium, and hair follicles, bear the brunt of the toxic effects of the anticancer drugs. Fortunately, the rapidly proliferating normal and cancer cells are not always equally vulnerable, and the principle of selective toxicity can be utilized. It is apparent, however, that the margin of safety is often a narrow one.

Resistance

The other factor that often limits the clinical usefulness of a chemotherapeutic agent is the emergence of a line of malignant cells resistant to the drug. It is a common clinical experience to find that the first trial of a given drug with a cancer patient is successful and that subsequent trials are often progressively less successful until no apparent beneficial effect is achieved by administering the drug.

Probably a number of cellular mechanisms are involved in drug resistance: altered metabolism of the drug, impermeability to the active compound, increased activity of an inhibited enzyme, increased cellular repair activity, and others. There is obviously an analogy between the development of resistance to drugs in cancer therapy and the appearance of drug-resistant strains of bacteria during the course of an infection. The approach of the clinician is the same in both situations—change drugs or, less often, use larger doses of the same drug.

Combinations of Agents

One recent approach to delaying the emergence of resistant malignant cell lines is the use of several drugs with different modes of action simultaneously (for example, see in Chapter 3 the discussion of combination therapy of testicular germinal cell neoplasms). Except in a few well-established situations, this approach with multiple agents is still experimental. The combining of chemotherapeutic agents is so logical that one wonders why it was not attempted earlier.

At the risk of oversimplification, it is helpful to think of a population of malignant cells as resembling a culture of bacteria. In both, combinations of agents can delay or suppress the emergence of drug-resistant cells and can prolong the time necessary for the population of malignant cells to reach a density that produces clinically apparent disease. Addition of an anticancer drug to malignant cells results in the killing of the drug-sensitive cells, just as addition of an antibiotic to bacteria results in the killing of bacteria. If the drug is not wholly effective, then a portion of the cancer (or bacterial population) survives.

The surviving population contains drug-resistant cells; these are the cells that have mechanisms for preventing entry of the drug or that have the ability to circumvent the drug's inhibitory effect on cellular metabolism. If these drug-resistant cells are capable of replication, they give rise to a drug-resistant tumor (or bacterial population). The administered drug thus has a selective mode of action leading to the emergence of a resistant cell line. The frequency of emergence of an antibiotic-resistant bacterium can be determined precisely. It is less easy to determine the frequency of occurrence of drug-resistant cancer cells. It is obvious, however, that the chances for the development of a drug-resistant line will not be as good if two or more drugs of dissimilar modes of action can be used in a treatment combination. This principle can be demonstrated by a simple example.

A patient with acute lymphocytic leukemia may have 10^{12} malignant cells in his body. If a single drug, for example, prednisone, is 99.999 per cent effective (i.e., if it kills 99,999 of every 100,000 tumor cells), then 10^7 malignant cells remain after prednisone therapy. If, in addition, a second agent with a different mode of action, such as vincristine, is 99.9 per cent effective, the population of malignant cells can be further reduced to 10^4. If still more agents are used, it is theoretically possible to reduce the cell population to zero. At present, this goal is not obtainable because of many factors: limitations imposed by toxicity to normal tissues are compounded by multiple agents; malignant cells are concentrated in sites not reached by the drug (e.g., the central nervous system); cells may be in a prolonged G1 or G0 phase and thus unaffected by cell cycle-specific agents.

Even though combinations of drugs may not eradicate all malignant cells and thus cure the patient of his disease, they certainly prolong the period of freedom from symptomatic disease.

CLASSES OF CHEMOTHERAPEUTIC AGENTS

Alkylating Agents

The commonly used alkylating agents include nitrogen mustard (HN_2, mechlorethamine hydrochloride, Mustargen), cyclophosphamide (Endoxan, Cytoxan), chlorambucil (Leukeran), melphalan (Alkeran), and busulfan (Myleran). Figure 2–1 shows the structure of

HN₂

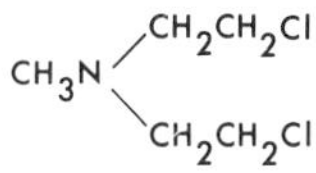

CH_3N $\diagup CH_2CH_2Cl$ $\diagdown CH_2CH_2Cl$

Methyl-bis (β-chloroethyl) amine

CHLORAMBUCIL

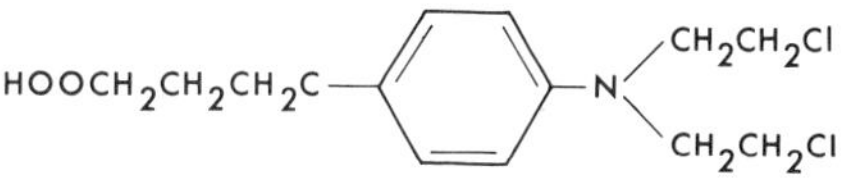

$HOOCH_2CH_2CH_2C$ — (ring) — $N \diagup CH_2CH_2Cl \diagdown CH_2CH_2Cl$

4-(p-[Bis(β-chloroethyl)amino]phenyl) butyric acid

MELPHALAN

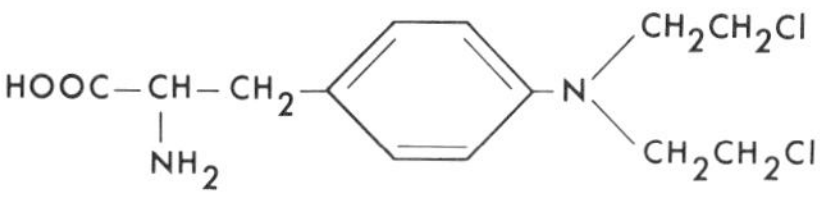

$HOOC-CH-CH_2$ — (ring) — $N \diagup CH_2CH_2Cl \diagdown CH_2CH_2Cl$
|
NH_2

p-Bis(β-chloroethyl)aminophenylalanine

CYCLOPHOSPHAMIDE

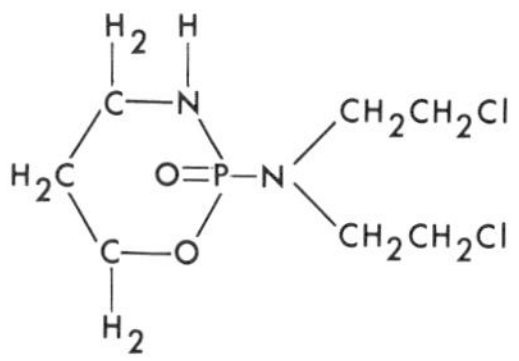

H_2C $C-N$ $O=P-N \diagup CH_2CH_2Cl \diagdown CH_2CH_2Cl$ $C-O$

2-[Bis(β-chloroethyl)amino] -2H-1,3,2-
oxazaphosphorinane, 2-oxide

BUSULFAN

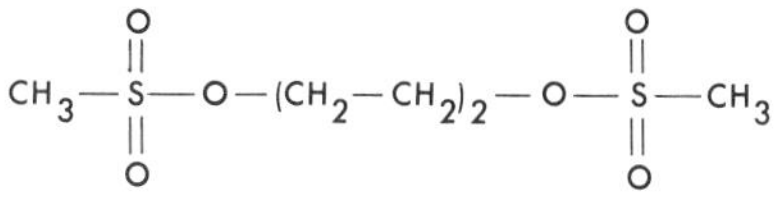

$CH_3-S-O-(CH_2-CH_2)_2-O-S-CH_3$

1,4-Dimethanesulfonoxybutane

Figure 2-1 Chemical structure of polyfunctional alkylating agents.

these compounds. The alkylating agents are extremely reactive compounds, which can substitute an alkyl group (for example, R-CH²-CH²-) for the hydrogen atoms of many organic compounds. Many cellular substances can be alkylated in this way. However, the preponderance of evidence suggests that it is the alkylation of nucleic acids — and primarily of DNA — that is critical to the cytotoxic effects of these compounds.[1,2] Such alkylation produces breaks in the DNA molecule and cross-linking of the twin strands of DNA, thus interfering with DNA replication and transcription of RNA. Similar effects are produced by certain kinds of ionizing radiation.[3,4] The alkylators are said to be "radiomimetic." The effects of alkylators, like the corresponding ones of x-rays, are often visible microscopically as abnormalities of chromosome structure.

There are two classes of alkylating agents, monofunctional and polyfunctional. The monofunctional compound has only one alkylating group; the polyfunctional compound has more than one. In general, the polyfunctional agents have proved to be more useful clinically. With one exception, the clinically useful alkylating agents are derivatives of nitrogen mustard (Fig. 2–1). The exception is busulfan, an alkyl sulfonate.

The differences in activity among the various alkylating agents are apparently related to differences in absorption, site and rate of metabolism, and tissue affinity rather than to a basic difference in mode of action. To paraphrase Gertrude Stein, "a mustard is a mustard is a mustard." Expressed less poetically, all mustards administered to the same level of toxicity produce similar antitumor effects. One's choice of alkylators, therefore, reflects certain clinical considerations, such as the route of administration, the desired rapidity of effect, the presence of bowel, hepatic, or genitourinary disease, and the experience of the therapist. For a detailed consideration of the mode of action of alkylating agents, the reader is referred to the excellent reviews of Wheeler,[1] Ochoa and Hirschberg,[4] and Calabresi and Welch.[5] A guide to the alkylating agents generally used is given in Table 2–1.

Alkylating agents appear to be cell cycle-nonspecific and are active against a wide range of tumors with differing rates of proliferation. There is considerable difference in sensitivity of different cell types to the cytotoxic effects of alkylating agents. The mammalian lymphocyte, despite its relatively low proliferative activity, is very sensitive to the effects of alkylating agents.

NITROGEN MUSTARD. Because nitrogen mustard is a vesicant, it must be given intravenously, care being taken that the preparation

TABLE 2–1 *Alkylating Agents*

Compound	Chemical Characteristics	Clinical Considerations	Route of Administration	Available Preparations
Nitrogen mustard (Mustargen)	Ethylamine	Rapidly acting; vesicant action	I.V.; intracavitary	Powder (unstable after hydration)
Cyclophosphamide (Cytoxan)	Phosphoric acid derivative of HN_2	Effective orally with slow onset; rapid I.V. effect; requires metabolism by liver; produces alopecia and cystitis	Oral; I.V.	50 mg. tablets; powder
Chlorambucil (Leukeran)	Phenylbutyric acid derivative of HN_2	Slow onset; usually easy to control	Oral	2 mg. tablets
Melphalan (Alkeran)	Phenylalanine derivative of HN_2	May have rapid effect and be difficult to control	Oral	2 mg. tablets
Busulfan (Myleran)	Alkyl sulfonate	Appears to be selectively myelosuppressive; effective in chronic myeloproliferative disorders; thrombocytopenia often difficult to manage	Oral	2 mg. tablets

does not infiltrate the soft tissues or even splash on the exposed skin or conjunctivae of the patient or physician. It is usually injected directly into intravenous tubing through which physiologic saline solution is running. Because of the severe nausea and vomiting invariably accompanying mustard administration, the patient is often given an antiemetic such as prochlorperazine (10 to 20 mg.) before administration of the alkylator. A sedative such as chloral hydrate (1 to 2 gm.) is often helpful in reducing untoward symptoms. Since the compound rapidly reacts with water and undergoes chemical transformation, it is prepared immediately before use. If there are any delays in its administration after hydration, it is likely that the compound will be inactive.

Nitrogen mustard rapidly interacts with cells in vivo, and it appears that its primary activity occurs within a few seconds or minutes; therefore, the only control the physician has over the drug is at the time of administration. He can vary the dose of mustard, but cannot otherwise titrate the drug, as he can the slower acting alkylating agents. This fact has led to some decrease in the use of nitrogen mustard in favor of other related compounds in recent years. Nitrogen mustard, however, is still a very useful drug when the physician desires a rapid cytotoxic effect and has experience in judging an effective dose. Nitrogen mustard is also useful for direct intracavitary injection in treating recalcitrant malignant effusions. When it is used in this manner, absorption of the mustard from the cavity may produce systemic effects.

The dosage of nitrogen mustard varies with the previous chemotherapeutic history and the related marrow reserve of the patient and, to some extent, with the type of malignancy being treated. In a previously untreated patient, a dosage of 0.5 mg. per kg. given in divided doses of 0.25 mg. per kg. on each of two successive days is usually sufficient. Dosages in excess of 0.6 mg. per kg. are dangerous; dosages as low as 0.2 mg. per kg. may suffice for chronic lymphocytic leukemia. For intracavitary administration the dosage is 0.2 to 0.4 mg./kg. If the patient has inadequate bone marrow reserves as reflected in a low white blood cell count or platelet count, or marrow hypoplasia, or abnormal stimulation tests,[6] a lower dose of mustard is given.

The nadir of the fall in white blood count and platelet count usually occurs within 7 to 21 days of injection. The patient should be followed closely at this time. The fall may be greater in a patient whose bone marrow has been damaged by previous chemotherapy, radiation therapy, or malignant infiltration. Infection and bleeding associated with bone marrow depression are the most serious toxic side effects of nitrogen mustard, although the acute gastrointestinal symptoms and later menstrual irregularities, and rarely alopecia, may be annoying to the patient. Obviously the drug should be used only if absolutely necessary in a pregnant patient. The white blood count and platelet count usually begin to rise by the second to fourth week after drug administration, but it is usually advisable to delay administration of a second course of the drug for at least six weeks.

Nitrogen mustard has a time-honored place in the treatment of disseminated Hodgkin's disease and other lymphomas, including mycosis fungoides. It may also be useful in occasional patients with carcinoma of the head and neck, breast, ovary, and lung. In general, it is not useful in treating the acute leukemias or multiple myeloma, and the slower acting alkylators are preferable in managing chronic lymphocytic leukemia. Nitrogen mustard is often used in conjunction with radiation therapy in the treatment of spinal cord compression secondary to lymphoma. This complication constitutes one of the few hematologic emergencies. In such a situation, if prompt initial chemotherapy is followed within a day or two by initiation of definitive radiation therapy, the neurologic lesion is often reversible.

CYCLOPHOSPHAMIDE.   This widely used alkylating agent is effective by both the oral and the intravenous routes of administration. Cyclophosphamide must be metabolized in vivo before it exerts cytotoxic effects.[7] Metabolism probably takes place mainly within the liver. This fact has certain clinical correlates. The drug is probably not directly effective by intracavitary administration; rather, its effect on malignant pleural effusions is via its systemic effect. This behavior is in contrast to that of nitrogen mustard. In theory, cyclophosphamide may have reduced effectiveness in patients with severe hepatocellular disease, although I know of no documentation of this situation.

Cyclophosphamide produces the toxicities in rapidly proliferating normal tissues in common with all of the clinically useful alkylating agents. The often-repeated statement that cyclophosphamide has a platelet-sparing effect[8] is not well substantiated and is probably unfounded. It is simply easier to control this orally effective, slowly acting alkylator, making it possible to avoid significant depression of thrombocytopoiesis. Large doses of cyclophosphamide produce thrombocytopenia in the same way nitrogen mustard does.

In addition to marrow suppression, cyclophosphamide has some other clinically important toxicities. Alopecia is a frequent side effect,[9] and it is often advisable to warn the female patient of this complication beforehand, in order that she prepare herself for this possibility and obtain a wig if necessary. Metabolites of cyclophosphamide are excreted in the urine, and the drug can produce severe hemorrhagic cystitis.[9, 10] In my own experience, this is almost always avoidable when a high fluid output is maintained. Dehydration must be avoided if this drug is used.

The usual oral dosage of cyclophosphamide is 1 to 2.5 mg. per kg. per day in divided doses. The best guides to regulating the oral dosage are the response of the disease and the level of the white blood count, which should be maintained at about 4000 per cu. mm. When a more rapid drug effect is desired, cyclophosphamide may be given intravenously in divided doses totaling 7 to 30 mg. per kg. over 2 to 4 days. Rarely 40 to 50 mg. per kg. is administered. The use of repeated courses is guided by the response of the tumor and the levels of the leukocyte and platelet counts. It is usually advisable to wait at least two weeks after a large intravenous dose before giving additional drug.

In general, intravenously administered cyclophosphamide is used in the same situations as nitrogen mustard. It is often effective in treating lymphomas and certain carcinomas. In addition, clinical experience has indicated that it may be effective in multiple myeloma and acute leukemia, especially acute lymphoblastic leukemia refractory to more usual therapy. The drug is usually given by the oral route in patients with these diseases. As a rule, cyclophosphamide is not effective in patients with lymphoma when the lesion has proved resistant to adequate doses of other alkylating agents.

CHLORAMBUCIL. Chlorambucil is probably the easiest alkylating agent to use. It is an aromatic derivative of nitrogen mustard that is effective by the oral route of administration. It is the slowest acting and generally least toxic of the alkylating agents in general use. If the drug is given for prolonged periods of time, it may produce myelosuppression, gastrointestinal symptoms, and, rarely, hepatotoxicity and dermatitis. These toxic side effects are usually avoidable if proper attention is paid to the patient and the laboratory studies.

Chlorambucil is frequently used in chronic lymphocytic leukemia to reduce the mass of abnormal lymphoid tissue and in lymphomas to induce or maintain a remission.[11, 12] The initial dosage is usually 0.1 mg. per kg. per day in either a single or divided doses. Once the desired effect is achieved, usually in 3 to 4 weeks, maintenance therapy with 2 to 4 mg. per day may be considered. It is important that maintenance dosage not exceed these levels, since it is far more difficult to treat aplastic anemia than the usual case of chronic lymphocytic leukemia. Chlorambucil, like other alkylators, has been used in the treatment of malignancies of the breast[13] and ovary.[14] Although it has also been used in treating patients with multiple myeloma, macroglobulinemia, choriocarcinoma, and testicular tumors, the general experience with this agent is less extensive than with other alkylators.

MELPHALAN. Melphalan is a phenylalanine derivative of nitrogen mustard that is generally given orally. A comprehensive review of melphalan and related compounds has been prepared by White.[15] Melphalan is probably the most difficult of the modern oral alkylating agents to use, myelosuppression being the chief toxic side effect. This drug has been used most extensively in the treatment of multiple myeloma, in which its effectiveness is roughly comparable to that of cyclophosphamide.[16, 17] Relatively little experience in treating other malignancies has been reported, and, in general, its use at present is restricted to patients with myeloma. It is usually given in a dosage of 0.05 to 0.1 mg. per kg. per day in divided doses until the leukocyte count is less than 4000 per cu. mm. or thrombocytopenia is observed. The drug is stopped until there is evidence of hematologic recovery and then is resumed at a maintenance level of 1 to 4 mg. per day. Therapy is usually continued intermittently for several months. The initial fall in the white cell count usually takes place 2 to 3 weeks after initiation of therapy, but in some patients it may occur as early as day 5; therefore, patients receiving this drug must be watched extremely carefully.

BUSULFAN.   This alkyl sulfonate is related to the mustards in its mechanism of action. Its predominant effect is against cells of the granulocytic series. Detailed pharmacokinetic studies of this compound have been performed in man.[18, 19] After intravenous administration of ^{14}C-labeled busulfan, the drug rapidly disappears from the circulation. Two major and 10 minor ^{14}C-containing metabolites have been isolated from the urine but not identified.

Busulfan is effective by the oral route and is widely used in the treatment of patients with chronic myelocytic leukemia and occasionally of patients with polycythemia and other myeloproliferative disorders. In the latter, the drug is usually restricted to those patients with myeloid metaplasia whose disease picture resembles chronic myelocytic leukemia, or to those patients with symptomatic essential thrombocytosis.

Busulfan is generally given in dosages of 4 to 10 mg. per day to patients with chronic myelocytic leukemia until the white blood cell count falls to the range of 10,000 to 15,000 per cu. mm.; it is then discontinued. Maintenance therapy is begun when the white count shows a tendency to rise above this range; the maintenance dosage is usually of the order of 2 to 4 mg. per day.

The proper use of busulfan requires experience, since it occasionally produces abrupt drops in the white blood count and platelet count, which may be irreversible. The acute toxicities of busulfan are almost exclusively hematopoietic. The major ones are suppression of platelet and granulocyte production. These may be delayed in appearance and make the determination of dosage difficult. With prolonged administration, complex and interesting side effects can occur, including hyperpigmentation resembling that of Addison's disease or porphyria cutanea tarda, pulmonary fibrosis, and gynecomastia.[20-22]

Antimetabolites

Hundreds of antimetabolites have been developed and tested in the last 15 years. Of this large group, only three agents have been adopted for general clinical use. These agents are methotrexate (Methotrexate), a folic acid antagonist; 6-mercaptopurine (6-MP, Purinethol), a purine analog; and 5-fluorouracil (5-FU, Fluorouracil), a pyrimidine analog (Fig. 2–2). Cytosine arabinoside (Ara-C, Cytarabine), a novel pyrimidine nucleoside analog, is not currently on the market for general use but almost certainly will soon be available. A guide to the use of these agents is summarized in Table 2–2.

METHOTREXATE. The development of folic acid antagonists followed (1) the characterization of the essential role of folic acid in proliferating cells synthesizing nucleic acid and nucleic acid precursors and (2) the observation that folic acid administration sometimes resulted in the exacerbation of acute leukemia. The introduction of methotrexate by Farber and his colleagues[23] in 1948 marked the beginning of an important new phase in the history of chemotherapy. Many folic acid analogs have been developed and used clinically, but the original compound, methotrexate, is still the best available agent in this group.

Folic acid coenzymes are involved in the synthesis of key precursors of nucleic acids and proteins and, as such, are critical to the metabolism of proliferating cells. In addition, they generally act as carriers of one-carbon units, although in some instances they may also

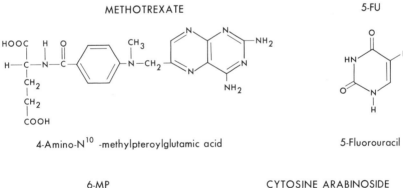

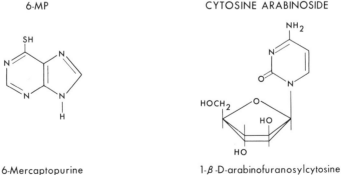

Figure 2–2   Chemical structure of antimetabolites.

TABLE 2-2 *Antimetabolites*

Compound	Chemical Characteristics	Clinical Considerations	Route of Administration	Available Preparations
Methotrexate	Folic acid antagonist	Renal excretion; absorbed from meningeal surfaces; toxicity for marrow, G.I. tract, and buccal mucosa; renal toxicity at high doses; hepatic toxicity with prolonged administration	Oral	2.5 mg. tablets; powder
6-Mercaptopurine (Purinethol)	Purine analog; the ribotide interferes with purine synthesis and interconversion	Xanthine oxidase metabolism and renal excretion; marrow and hepatic toxicity	Oral; I.V. (rare)	50 mg. tablets
5-Fluorouracil (Fluorouracil)	Fluoropyrimidine; interferes with DNA synthesis via the thymidylate synthetase reaction	Hepatic metabolism; marrow and G.I. toxicity frequent	I.V. only	500 mg. in 10 ml.
Cytosine arabinoside	Pyrimidine nucleoside analog with an altered sugar moiety	Rapidly excreted in urine	I.V.	Not generally available

participate in the oxidoreduction of one-carbon units.[24] The enzyme dihydrofolate reductase appears to be the principal focus of attack of the folic acid antagonists. This enzyme is involved in the synthesis of tetrahydrofolate, one of the active forms of the coenzyme. The effective folate antagonists such as methotrexate are bound very strongly to this enzyme, so strongly that the interaction was first thought to be irreversible.[25]

These observations have relevance for the clinician. If an overdose of methotrexate is given, toxicity may persist for some time. For the first few minutes or hours after an overdose, a biologically active form of folic acid (such as folinic acid) may prevent side effects; forms of folic acid that require conversion to the tetrahydroform will be ineffective in treating toxicity. After the first few hours, even biologically active folate coenzymes will be of no avail, since the major damage to proliferating cells will have been done.

Proliferating bone marrow cells, skin, and gastrointestinal epithelium cells are the principal targets of toxicity. The buccal mucosa is particularly vulnerable. At high doses, methotrexate can produce renal injury.[26] With prolonged administration of this drug, cirrhosis and portal hypertension can occur.[27]

When given intrathecally, the drug is readily absorbed from the subarachnoid space and may produce systemic toxicity; therefore, all systemic therapy is usually stopped for a few days at the time of intrathecal treatment. From 50 to 90 per cent of administered methotrexate is rapidly excreted in the urine. If standard doses of methotrexate are given to patients with impaired renal function, prolonged high blood and tissue levels of the drug produce severe toxicity. Therefore, smaller than normal doses are given to patients with diminished renal function.

We probably know more about the development of cell lines resistant to methotrexate than we do of acquired resistance to any other chemotherapeutic agent. Probable mechanisms of the development of resistance include increased levels of dihydrofolate reductase and production of an altered enzyme with decreased affinity for the drug.[28] Decreased rates of entry of the drug into the tumor cell and increased levels of drug-metabolizing enzymes (e.g., aldehyde oxidase) are other possible mechanisms of acquired resistance.[29]

Methotrexate finds its major use in the treatment of acute leukemia, in both systemic and meningeal forms. It is also useful in treating patients with choriocarcinoma and some patients with mycosis fungoides, carcinoma of the breast, carcinoma of the head and neck, and carcinoma of the lung. Except in the treatment of acute leukemia, no uniform, widely accepted dosage schedule for methotrexate has been agreed upon. Even in the case of acute leukemia, an optimal dosage schedule has not been determined. For the treatment of particular malignancies with methotrexate, the appropriate chapters should be consulted.

The conventional dosage of methotrexate in acute leukemia has been 3 mg./sq. M./day, or approximately 5 mg. per day by mouth in adults. Recently the concept has emerged that in this disease methotrexate should be given in intensive courses with larger doses, until the emergence of toxic side effects requires reduction or withdrawal of the drug (cf. ref. 30). Dosages up to 10 mg. per kg. per day have been given intravenously in short courses.

Methotrexate has an important place in the treatment of meningeal leukemia, a clinical complication that usually occurs in the course of acute lymphoblastic leukemia. In the treatment of meningeal leukemia, methotrexate is usually injected into the lumbar subarachnoid space in a dose of 5 to 10 mg. dissolved in 10 to 15 ml. of saline. To assure complete distribution of the drug, barbotage may be used. Intrathecally administered courses may be repeated every other day or weekly until evidence of leukemic involvement disappears or toxicity intervenes. It is important to realize that methotrexate is readily absorbed from the meninges and may produce systemic toxicity. Therefore, systemic therapy is usually discontinued at the time of intrathecal administration. Alternatively, citrovorum factor (folinic acid, a biologically active form of folic acid) can be given intravenously in a dose of 3 to 10 mg. at the same time that methotrexate is given intrathecally. Several good reviews of the biochemistry and pharmacology of folic acid antagonists have recently been published.[31–32]

6-MERCAPTOPURINE.   6-Mercaptopurine (6-MP) is a purine analog used chiefly in the treatment of acute leukemia (Fig. 2–2). Its discovery by Elion, Burge, and Hitchings[33] in 1952 followed the investigations of Hitchings and his collaborators, begun in the early 1940's. 6-MP must be converted to the ribonucleotide before it can act as an effective inhibitor of purine biosynthesis. One mechanism of acquired drug resistance by certain cell lines may be the failure to convert 6-MP to the active ribonucleotide form. In the form of the ribonucleotide the two major effects of 6-MP appear to be (1) interference with de novo purine biosynthesis from small precursors (inosinic acid is the first purine-containing compound to be formed in the de novo pathway) and (2) interference with the interconversions of purines, and especially with the formation of adenylic and guanylic acid from inosinic acid.

A number of purine analogs have been developed and tested. Several are effective, but to date none has demonstrated clear superiority over 6-MP for clinical usefulness. The reader is referred to the excellent reviews by Elion, Hitchings, and their colleagues[33-36] and by Calabresi and Welch[5] for a complete summary of 6-MP metabolism and its mode of action.

In the use of 6-MP two points are worth stressing. The first is that the effects of the drug may be delayed for several weeks. Although a response to 6-MP may be observed within one week after the beginning of therapy, it is often delayed for three and even four weeks. The second point is that cross-resistance between 6-MP and other clinically useful anticancer drugs (exclusive of purine analogs) does not occur.

6-MP is readily absorbed by the intestinal epithelium and is rapidly catabolized and excreted in the urine. It does not readily cross the blood-brain barrier and consequently is not useful in the treatment of meningeal leukemia. The pharmacokinetics of this drug have recently been described in detail.[37]

A major metabolic pathway of 6-MP catabolism to 6-thiouric acid is mediated by xanthine oxidase enzymes. The widely used xanthine oxidase inhibitor, allopurinol, delays metabolism of 6-MP and increases its clinical potency twofold to fourfold. Therefore, the daily dosage of 6-MP should be reduced to one-quarter or one-half the usual dosage when allopurinol is administered at a daily dosage of 300 to 600 mg.

The principal toxicities of 6-MP are associated with marrow injury, but the drug can also cause jaundice, which is apparently related to cholestasis and to hepatocellular injuries.[38, 39] Jaundice usually clears with drug withdrawal. Hyperuricemia is a frequent complication of 6-MP treatment. Allopurinol, in a dosage of 300 to 400 mg. per day, in combination with a high urine output, will usually suffice to prevent this complication. Dermatitis is a rare complication of 6-MP treatment.

In the therapy of acute leukemia, 6-MP is better as a remission-maintaining agent than as a remission-inducing agent. It is often used to maintain a remission in a patient with acute lymphoblastic leukemia. In this situation the drug is generally administered orally, 1.5 to 2.5 mg. per kg. per day, in divided doses. The exact level of drug is usually determined by the level of the white blood count. The appearance of hypersegmented neutrophils in the peripheral blood smear is often an early warning of emergent drug toxicity. Determinations should also be made of the serum bilirubin, hepato-cellular enzymes such as serum glutamic-oxaloacetic transaminase, and serum alkaline phosphatase during 6-MP treatment. It is prob-able that the drug should be used in smaller than usual doses in patients with impaired renal function.

6-MP is also used in combination with other drugs to induce a remission in acute lymphoblastic leukemia; in this situation it is usually given in short five-day courses at three to five times the usual dose level. 6-MP has been used alone in attempts to induce remis-sions in acute myelocytic or myelomonocytic leukemia. In these diseases this drug has been only rarely effective, and superior thera-peutic regimens have recently been described.

6-MP is occasionally used in the treatment of chronic myelocytic leukemia when it has become refractory to busulfan. In general, however, 6-MP is a clearly inferior drug against this chronic condi-tion. 6-MP has been used experimentally in idiopathic thrombocyto-penic purpura and "autoimmune" hemolytic anemias resistant to standard therapy. There is as yet no convincing evidence for the general effectiveness of 6-MP in treating these diseases.

5-FLUOROURACIL. 5-Fluorouracil (5-FU) was developed by Heidelberger and his colleagues in 1957 on the basis of a rational biochemical approach to the treatment of malignant disease. Their subsequent five-year experience is summarized in reference 40. 5-FU is an analog of thymine (5-methyl uracil), one of the pyrimidine bases occurring in DNA but not in RNA (Fig. 2–2). The usefulness of 5-FU was predicated on the basis of possible interference with the sequence of reactions terminating in the biosynthesis of the deoxyri-bonucleotide of thymine (thymidylic acid). These predictions regard-ing 5-FU were amply confirmed by subsequent experience.[40]

There is still controversy as to the sites of 5-FU activity within the cell. It seems likely, however, that its principal effect is exerted by interference with thymidylate synthetase, the enzyme necessary to form thymidylic acid, a DNA precursor.[41] This interference is demonstrable only after 5-FU is converted to the deoxyribonucleotide. Fluorouracil is also converted to the ribonucleotide and, as such, interferes with RNA synthesis. This is thought to be an undesirable feature of the drug, since it results in less specificity for neoplastic cells. An analog of 5-FU, 5-fluorouracil deoxyribonucleoside, has some theoretical advantages over the parent compound, but at the present time has no demonstrable practical advantages.

5-FU appears to be metabolized principally by the liver. Only a small fraction of the drug appears in the urine. If it is given orally, the drug's route to the liver via the portal circulation results in catabolism and variable clinical effectiveness. Therefore, the drug is usually given intravenously by rapid injection or slow infusion.[42]

The principal toxicities of 5-FU are observed in the bone marrow and gastrointestinal epithelium. Megaloblastic changes are an early sign of toxicity, and complete marrow aplasia is a late manifestation. Ulcerations of the buccal mucosa, nausea, anorexia, and diarrhea are common complaints of patients receiving this drug. The usual sequence of events visible to the physician is erythema of the buccal mucosa followed by development of a patchy white membrane and then ulceration. These toxicities are the usual factors limiting drug administration. In addition, alopecia, hyperpigmentation, and skin atrophy have occasionally been reported, and neuropathic toxicities, including myelopathy, have occurred.

5-Fluorouracil may be difficult to use because of its propensity to produce severe, life-threatening depression of the bone marrow. It should not be given without extremely close supervision of the patient and his hematologic status. This is particularly true in a patient with a limited bone marrow reserve either from previous therapy or from malignant involvement of the marrow. Since this drug depends on the liver for catabolism, a "standard" dose of 5-FU may also produce severe toxicity in the patient with impaired hepatocellular function.

At the present time 5-FU is most useful in the treatment of patients with carcinoma of the breast and gastrointestinal tract. The drug has also benefited occasional patients with carcinoma of the cervix or ovary, although objective antitumor responses, usually lasting less than six months, are realized in only a minority of patients treated.

The optimal dosage for 5-FU has yet to be established. Much effort has already been expended in trials of modifications of the "standard" course in order to reduce toxicity without sacrificing the drug's antitumor effect. One modification tested recently in protocol studies of the Western Cooperative Cancer Chemotherapy Group (WCCCG) has been reported by Jacobs et al.[42a] at the Cancer Research Institute at the University of California San Francisco Medical Center. It was found that a significant response rate could be obtained by adjusting the course to weekly rapid intravenous injections, without a loading dose. By the scheduling employed, doses were titrated to avoid major toxicity and drug-related deaths, and patients could be treated on an ambulatory basis. The dosage for the first four weeks was 15 mg. per kg. per week; this was increased to 20 mg. per kg. per week, if necessary, thereafter. An adequate course was considered to be one producing either an objective antitumor response or mild toxicity. If toxicity supervened, the 5-FU was stopped until symptoms had subsided and was then resumed at a dosage lower by 5 mg. per kg. In general, this modification has been associated with less drug toxicity than that encountered with the previously used standard course: intravenous injection of 15 mg. per kg. daily for 3 to 5 days and 7.5 mg. per kg. every 2 or 3 days to toxicity, repeated monthly.[43] Maximal white blood count depression usually occurs within 10 to 14 days after such a course.

At the moment, there is not enough evidence to warrant a firm statement about the value of maintenance therapy with 5-FU after an antitumor effect has been achieved. Our practice has been to continue weekly treatment of patients with carcinoma of the breast at drug levels that do not produce leukopenia. However, a study comparing the effectiveness of intermittent vs. maintenance therapy is still necessary.

CYTOSINE ARABINOSIDE.   Cytosine arabinoside (1-β-D-arabino-furanosylcytoside) is a relatively new chemotherapeutic agent.[44] It is included here because of its usefulness in the treatment of acute leukemia[45] and certain cases of disseminated lymphoma resistant to more standard therapy. Almost certainly this compound will soon be available for general use by physicians. Cytosine arabinoside is unique among the clinically useful purine and pyrimidine analogs in that the chemical modification is in the sugar moiety of the ribonucleoside rather than in the purine base itself. Cytosine arabinoside appears to work by inhibition of DNA synthesis at the level of the conversion of the ribose moiety of cytosine ribonucleoside diphosphate to the deoxyribose. Cytosine arabinoside thus inhibits synthesis of one of the critical building blocks of DNA.

The observed toxicities of this compound are directed at the rapidly proliferating tissues of the bone marrow and gastrointestinal tract. Gastrointestinal symptomatology has, in general, posed a principal limitation to treatment.

Cytosine arabinoside thus far has been used mainly in the treatment of acute myelocytic and myelomonocytic leukemia of adults. Its use in these diseases is still experimental and the optimal dosage schedule is still being determined. The compound appears to be rapidly excreted in the urine. Consequently, slow infusion over 8 to 12 hours appears to be more effective for a given dose than is rapid intravenous infusion. At present, daily infusion (over 8 hours) of 5 to 7.5 mg. per kg. repeated on each of 4 or 5 days appears to be an effective way of administering this compound. However, this may not be an optimal regimen and may be modified in the future. Such courses may be repeated until a remission occurs or toxicity prevents further therapy. Toxic depression of normal leukopoiesis and thrombopoiesis may appear within 14 days after the initial course of therapy. Several good reviews of the pharmacology and clinical use of this interesting compound are available.[46–48]

Antibiotics

Only one member of this class, actinomycin-D, has achieved the status of being a widely used drug (Table 2–3 and Figure 2–3). However, several others appear to be promising agents for the treatment of certain malignancies. Examples are mitomycin-C, mithramycin, and daunomycin. These antibiotics are natural products of certain soil fungi. They produce their antibiotic and tumoricidal effects by forming relatively stable complexes with DNA, thereby inhibiting synthesis of both DNA and RNA. They appear to be cell cycle-nonspecific agents, active at many stages within the cell replication cycle. Many of these compounds are light-sensitive and must be protected from light to avoid loss of activity.

ACTINOMYCIN-D. Actinomycin-D (Dactinomycin), the oldest and best known of the antitumor antibiotics, is widely used in the treatment of certain tumors of childhood, certain testicular tumors, and of choriocarcinoma. It was first isolated by Waksman and Woodruff in 1940 from *Streptomyces*.[49] Its mechanism of action at a molecular level has been well defined.[50] At relatively low concentrations in mammalian tissues, actinomycin-D inhibits the RNA polymerase reaction by forming complexes with the guanine residues of DNA. At higher concentrations it also inhibits DNA synthesis. Failure of the antibiotic to enter malignant cells may be one mechanism of development of drug resistance.[51]

Actinomycin-D must be administered intravenously because of its erratic absorption if given orally. It is rapidly cleared from the circulation after intravenous injection, and roughly 10 per cent is

TABLE 2–3   *Antibiotics and Vinca Alkaloids*

COMPOUND	ORIGIN	CLINICAL CONSIDERATIONS	ROUTE OF ADMINIS-TRATION	AVAILABLE PREPA-RATIONS
Actinomycin-D (Dactinomycin)	*Streptomyces*	Hematopoietic and G. I. toxicity; locally irritating	I.V.	Powder, 500 μg./vial
Vincristine (Oncovin)	Plant alkaloid	Neurotoxicity; severe constipation	I.V.	Powder, 1 and 5 mg./vial
Vinblastine (Velban)	Plant alkaloid	Bone marrow toxicity	I.V.	Powder, 10 mg./vial

ACTINOMYCIN-D

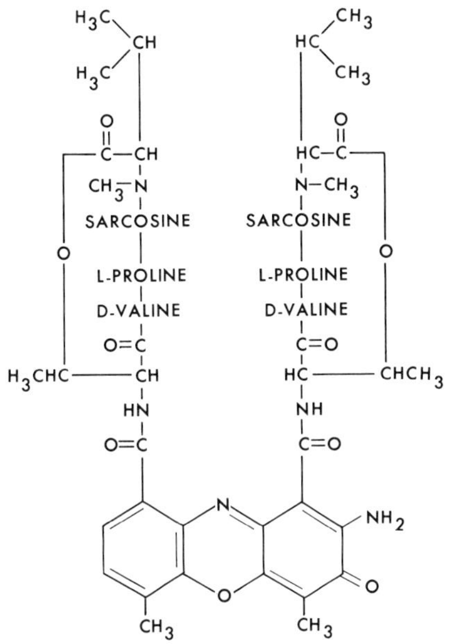

VINCA ALKALOIDS
VINCRISTINE
VINBLASTINE

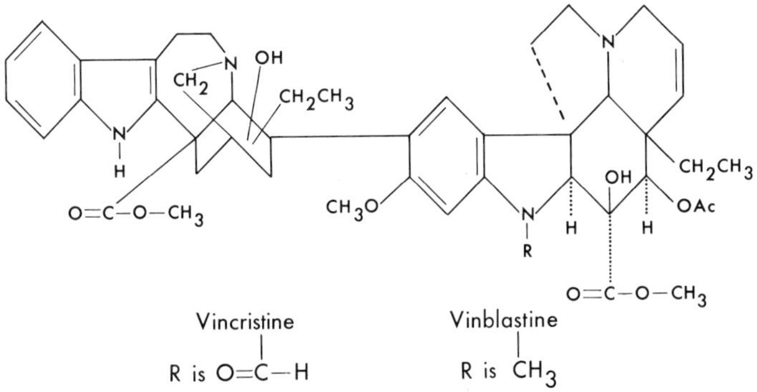

Vincristine

R is O=C—H

Vinblastine

R is CH₃

Figure 2–3 Chemical structure of antibiotics and plant alkaloids.

excreted unchanged in the urine and 50 per cent in the bile. Its primary toxicities are hematopoietic and gastrointestinal, including diarrhea, proctitis, and glossitis. Hematologic depression is usually apparent within 2 to 8 days after completion of a course of treatment. Local infiltration of the tissues with actinomycin-D produces local inflammation and necrosis. Consequently, the drug should be carefully injected into the tubing of an intravenous infusion to avoid extravasation.

A number of dosage regimens have been used, and the optimal program is still not known. At the University of California San Francisco Medical Center, for example, the usual dose of actinomycin-D is 15 μg. per kg. on each of 5 successive days, for a total dosage of 75 μg. per kg. Such a course may be repeated within 2 to 4 weeks. Lesser doses are used in treating adults if impaired marrow function is present and in treating small infants.

Mithramycin[52] and daunomycin[53] are promising new antibiotics with antitumor effects. These compounds are considered briefly in Chapters 3 and 10.

Vinca Alkaloids

The alkaloids vincristine (Oncovin) and vinblastine (Velban) have only recently been introduced for use by the chemotherapist (Table 2–3 and Fig. 2–3). These alkaloids, extracted from a variety of the periwinkle plant (*Vinca rosea Linn.*), have an interesting history. They were originally screened by American pharmaceutical houses because of their use as hypoglycemic agents by natives in several parts of the world. Their hypoglycemic properties were not very impressive; however, their marrow-depressant and other cytotoxic effects were readily apparent. As a consequence of this initial screening, these compounds underwent subsequent trials and eventually found a place as useful agents in cancer therapy.

The vinca alkaloids are large and complex molecules.[54] Vincristine and vinblastine differ only in having methyl (vinblastine) or formyl (vincristine) side chains on a large parent molecule. Despite this apparently minor chemical difference between these two molecules, they differ in their antitumor spectra and have widely different clinical toxicities.

The mode of antitumor action of these compounds is not known, although their many effects on cellular metabolism in vivo and in vitro are known.[55-57] They are mitotic inhibitors and mitotic poisons, and have complex effects on the synthesis of nucleic acids and proteins. In vitro, vincristine is active at extremely low concentrations (10^{-9}M or 10^{-10}M), a phenomenon which correlates with the low doses effective clinically (as little as 10 μg. per kg.).

At present, vinblastine is used mainly in the treatment of Hodgkin's disease and other lymphomas and of histiocytosis X and other reticuloendothelial malignancies of childhood. Vincristine is used in these diseases and, in addition, it is effective in the treatment of acute lymphoblastic leukemia and choriocarcinoma. Both drugs have been used in combination with other agents in experimental protocols in treating acute leukemia and certain solid tumors.

The principal clinical toxicity of vinblastine is bone marrow depression, particularly of the megakaryocytes and granulocytic

series. Vincristine, except at very high doses, has a relative granulo-
cyte-sparing effect. Its principal toxicity is neurologic. Unless carefully titrated, it produces both peripheral nervous system neuropathic
changes (mixed sensory and motor) and autonomic nervous neuro-
muscular toxicity. The latter may result in severe constipation and
even in bowel obstruction.

The early clues to the diagnosis of vincristine-induced neurotoxicity are numbness and paresthesia in the extremities and a loss of
the Achilles tendon reflexes. The bowel problems can usually be
prevented by the use of stool-softening agents and cathartics. It is
wise to avoid vincristine-induced neuropathic changes, which are
reversed only slowly or not at all after withdrawal of therapy. This
neurotoxicity may be associated with inappropriate antidiuretic hormone secretion.[58]

Vincristine and vinblastine are usually administered intravenously because of their unpredictable absorption when given orally.
Both compounds produce local damage if extravasated into the
tissues. Consequently, they are injected into intravenous tubing or
through a well-placed needle. Metabolism of these vinca alkaloids
appears to be primarily hepatic and less than 5 per cent appears in
the urine. Both vincristine and vinblastine are rapidly cleared from
the blood after intravenous injection.

The usual dose of vinblastine in treating disseminated lymphomas or reticuloendothelial malignancies is 0.1 to 0.15 mg. per kg.
given once in a 5- to 7-day period until the desired effect is achieved
or marrow depression precludes further therapy. Vincristine is given
to patients with lymphoma in weekly doses of 12.5 to 25 μg. per kg.
Such therapy may be continued for months and even years to maintain a patient in clinical remission. Somewhat higher doses (up to 75
μg. per kg.) are given to patients with acute leukemia and, in experimental protocols, in combination with other agents. This drug is
useful in induction of remission of acute leukemia, particularly
lymphoblastic, but is not very effective in maintaining a remission.
Consequently, in acute leukemia, the minimal dose of vincristine
necessary to achieve remission is used, and therapy with other
agents is then substituted.

Methylhydrazine Derivatives

Procarbazine (Natulan, Matulane, N-isopropyl-α-2-methylhydra-
zine) is a drug belonging to a new class of antineoplastic agents that
has recently become available for general use. (See Figure 2–4 and
Table 2–4.)

In preclinical studies, procarbazine was shown to possess a variety of biologic effects, including immunosuppression,[67] teratogen-
esis,[68] carcinogenesis,[69] cytotoxicity with mitotic suppression and

TABLE 2-4 *Methylhydrazine Derivatives*

COMPOUND	CHEMICAL CHARACTERISTICS	CLINICAL CONSIDERATIONS	ROUTE OF ADMINIS- TRATION	AVAILABLE PREPA- RATIONS
Procarbazine (Matulane)	Isopropyl- methylhydrazine	Marrow depression, central nervous system toxicity, monoamine oxidase inhibitor, hemolytic anemia	Oral	Capsules, 50 mg.

chromatin derangements,[70] and profound antineoplastic effects against a spectrum of transplanted tumors of mice and rats.[71]

Procarbazine has been employed in clinical investigation in Europe since 1962, and several hundreds of patients have since been treated. The most striking clinical responses have been seen in the lymphomas and especially Hodgkin's disease. In these studies no cross-resistance with other chemotherapeutic agents or with radiation therapy was demonstrable. A report in the American literature describes essentially similar findings.[72] The overall response rate is about 50 per cent; this includes both objective regression of disease and subjective clinical improvement.

When the drug is administered intravenously, there is rapid equilibration between plasma and cerebrospinal fluid. The biologic half-time of the drug is approximately 4 to 6 hours, and the major portion is excreted in the urine as N-isopropylterephthalamic acid. The mode of cytotoxic action of this drug is not clearly understood, but it has been suggested that the drug undergoes auto-oxidation with generation of hydrogen peroxide. The hydrogen peroxide then interacts directly with DNA in a manner presumed to be analogous to that of ionizing irradiation.

The toxic effects of procarbazine in man have included nausea and vomiting, marrow depression, central nervous system toxicity, dermatitis, and alopecia. The onset and duration of leukopenia and thrombocytopenia do not appear to be directly related to the total dose of drug. Methylhydrazine is a weak monoamine oxidase inhibitor. Such foods as ripe cheese and bananas, which have a high tyramine

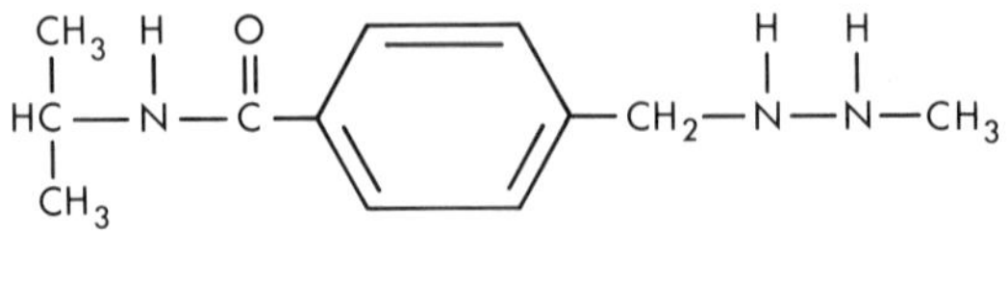

Procarbazine
Figure 2-4 Chemical structure of procarbazine.

content, should be avoided. Sympathomimetic drugs and tricyclic antidepressant drugs (e.g., imipramine) should be used with caution when procarbazine is administered concurrently.

At high dosage levels procarbazine produces somnolence and ataxia. Synergism between the sedative effects of methylhydrazine and phenothiazine derivatives have been apparent in some patients. To minimize central nervous system depression, barbiturates, narcotics, antihistamines, and sedative antihypotensive drugs should be used with caution in patients receiving procarbazine. Another pharmacologic incompatibility appears to be that with alcohol, and Antabuse-like reactions have been described.

In common with other hydrazine derivatives, procarbazine may produce hemolytic anemia with hemoglobin denaturation and the formation of Heinz bodies in red blood cells. These inclusions are made visible by supravital stains.

The procarbazine dosage should be reduced in patients with impaired hepatic or renal function or in those with damaged or replaced bone marrow.

The dosage of procarbazine in adults is generally 100 to 200 mg. daily by mouth for the first week. If the dosage is tolerated (i.e., no excessive gastrointestinal, hematopoietic, or central nervous system toxic effects), then the daily dosage is increased to 300 mg. The drug is continued at this level until the white blood count falls below 4000 per cu. mm. or the platelet count falls below 100,000 per cu. mm. The drug is then discontinued and is only resumed at reduced levels (50 to 100 mg. per day) when there is evidence of hematologic recovery.

Hormones

ESTROGENS.   The pioneering work of Huggins and his collaborators[59] in the early 1940's led to the development of androgen-control regimens for carcinoma of the prostate and paved the way for the modern era of rational cancer chemotherapy. Shortly thereafter, the results of estrogen treatment of carcinoma of the breast were reported in Great Britain and the United States.[60]

A vast number of estrogen analogs have been developed and given clinical trials.[61] It is safe to say that diethylstilbestrol, one of the earliest nonsteroidal estrogens introduced,[62] is still the compound of choice in cancer chemotherapy (Fig. 2–5). It is potent, inexpensive, and effective by oral administration and has a clinically satisfactory duration of action. It is clearly superior to any of the naturally occurring estrogens. Diethylstilbestrol, like many of the other nonsteroidal estrogens, is readily absorbed through skin, mucous membranes, and gastrointestinal epithelium. It is slowly de-

TESTOSTERONE PROPIONATE

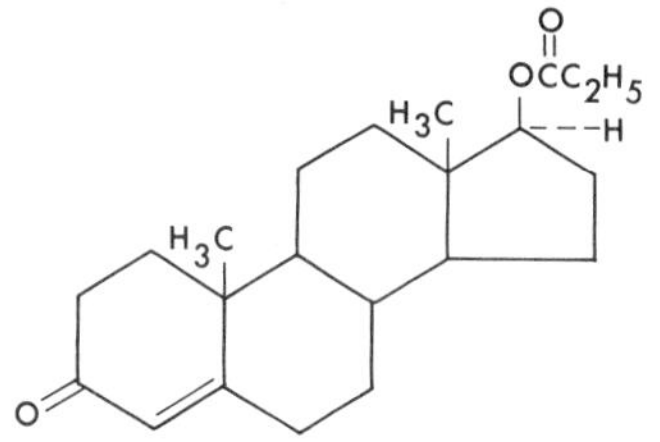

Δ^4-Androstene-17β-propionate-3-one

FLUOXYMESTERONE

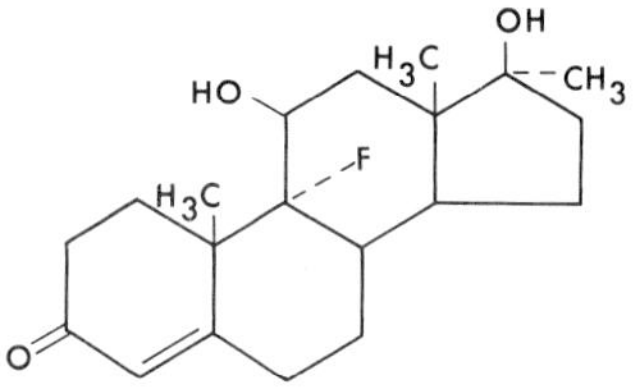

9α-Fluoro-11β-hydroxy-17α-
methyltestosterone

DIETHYLSTILBESTROL

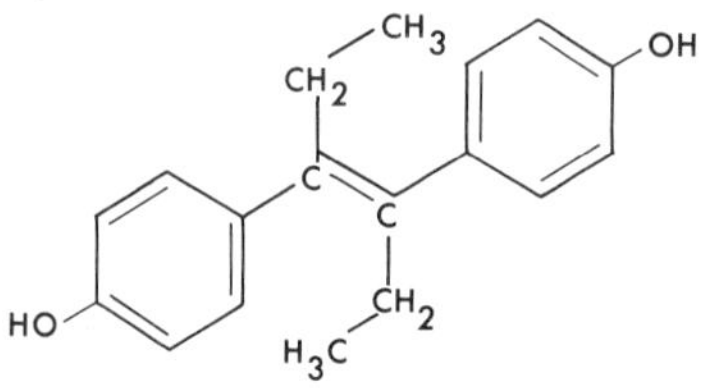

α,α'-Diethyl-4,4'-stilbenediol

PREDNISONE

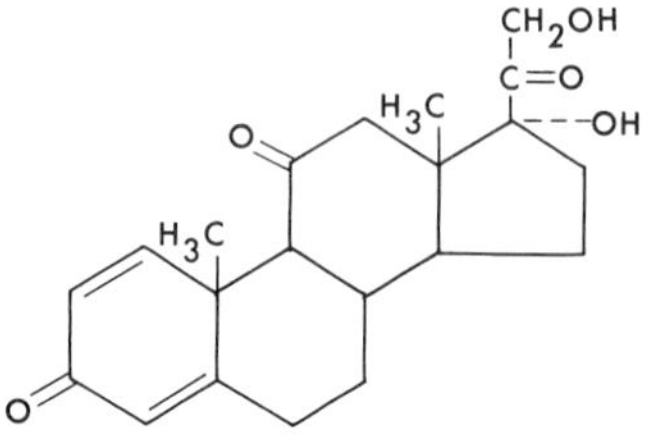

$\Delta^{1,4}$-Pregnadiene-17α, 21-diol-3, 11, 20-trione

17-HYDROXYPROGESTERONE CAPROATE

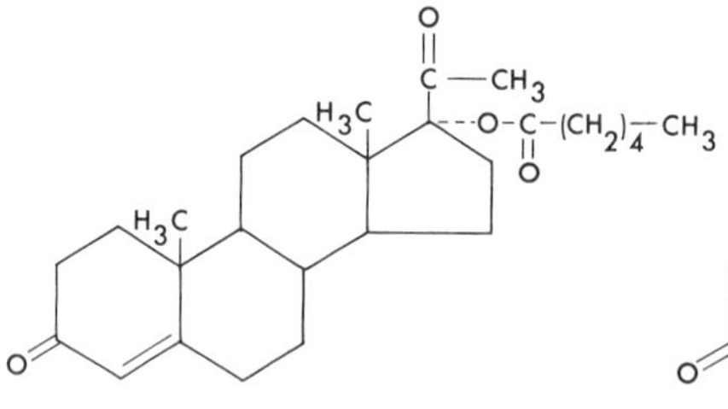

17α-Hydroxyprogesterone caproate

17-HYDROXY-6-METHYLPROGESTERONE

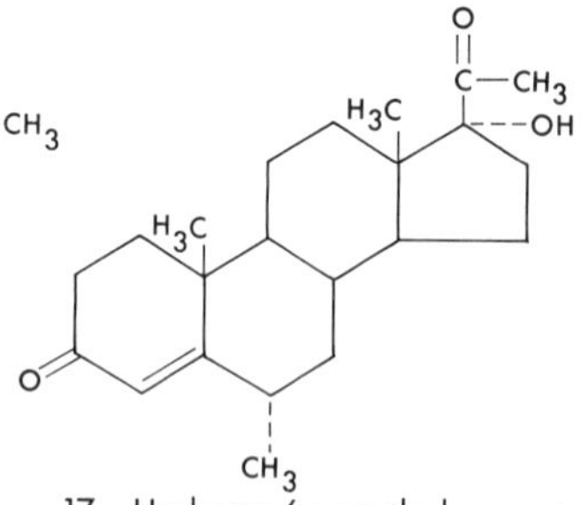

17α-Hydroxy-6α-methylprogesterone

Figure 2–5   Chemical structure of steroid compounds.

graded in the body. The precise pathway of its metabolism and excretion is poorly understood.

Tablets of diethylstilbestrol are available in doses of 0.1 to 25 mg. (Table 2–5). Because of its long duration of action, a single daily dose often suffices. The usual dose of diethylstilbestrol in carcinoma of the prostate is 1 to 3 mg. per day. Higher doses are occasionally needed in advanced disease. The most frequent undesirable side effects of estrogen therapy are gastrointestinal disturbances with nausea and vomiting. The symptoms often disappear despite continued treatment. Fluid retention in patients with cardiac, liver, or renal disease is another possible complication of therapy. Gynecomastia and changes in libido are occasional complications.

PROGESTATIONAL AGENTS. The major place of progestational agents in cancer chemotherapy has been in the treatment of patients with endometrial carcinoma. The use of these agents is usually restricted to patients with disseminated disease or patients in whom surgery and radiotherapy (the primary modalities of treatment) have failed or can no longer be used. These agents are also used occasionally in the treatment of patients with hypernephroma.

The naturally occurring progestins (e.g., progesterone) have no

TABLE 2–5 *Antitumor Hormones*

COMPOUND	CHEMICAL CHARACTERISTICS	CLINICAL CONSIDERATIONS	ROUTE OF ADMINISTRATION	AVAILABLE PREPARATIONS
Estrogen				
Diethylstilbestrol	Nonsteroidal estrogen	Potent estrogen; active by mouth; slow degradation; fluid retention and G.I. disturbances; feminization; uterine bleeding	Oral	Tablets, 0.1–25 mg.
Steroid Compounds				
Progestins				
Hydroxyprogesterone caproate (Delalutin)	Progestin	Minimal fluid retention; changes in epithelium of female genital tract and acinar cells of breast	I.M.	In oil, 125 and 250 mg./ml.
Medroxyprogesterone acetate (Depo-Provera)	Progestin	Fluid retention; changes in epithelial and acinar cells	I.M.	Suspension, 50 mg./ml.; 2.5 and 10 mg. tablets
Provera)			Oral	2.5 and 10 mg. tablets
Androgens				
Testosterone propionate (Perandren)	Testosterone ester	Virilization, fluid retention, change in libido	I.M.	In oil, 25 and 50 mg./ml.
Testosterone enanthate (Delatestryl)	Testosterone ester	Same	I.M.	In oil, 200 mg./ml.
Testosterone cypionate (Depo-testosterone)	Testosterone ester	Same	I.M.	In oil, 50, 100, and 200 mg./ml.
Fluoxymesterone (Halotestin)	Halogenated derivative	Same, plus oral absorption and hepatic toxicity	Oral	Tablets, 2, 5, and 10 mg.
Corticosteroids				
Prednisone	Synthetic analog of adrenal cortical steroid	Undesirable side effects: potassium loss, sodium and fluid retention, diabetes mellitus, psychosis, gastric bleeding	Oral	Tablets, 1, 2.5, 5, and 20 mg.

place in modern chemotherapy, and attention has been directed to synthetic compounds with a longer duration of action that are, in some cases, effective by mouth.[61] For obvious reasons, progestins with significant androgenic activity are undesirable. A number of agents with primary progestational activity and minimal androgenic and fluid-retaining effects are available, including medroxyprogesterone acetate (Provera) and hydroxyprogesterone caproate (Delalutin) (Table 2–5). Of these, hydroxyprogesterone caproate appears to be singularly free of fluid-retaining properties and has been most widely used in the treatment of endometrial carcinoma (Fig. 2–5). This drug is usually given intramuscularly in doses of 1 gm. twice weekly, or as much as 5 gm. weekly. All these progestins produce the typical progestational changes in the epithelium of the female genital tract and the acinar cells of the breast. Their precise mode of metabolism is not known. Progesterone, the parent compound, is catabolized largely in the liver, and its products are excreted in the urine.

Steroid Compounds

ANDROGENS. The principal place of androgens in the armamentarium of the chemotherapist is in the treatment of advanced carcinoma of the breast. Androgenic therapy for this condition has been used for about 30 years.[61, 63] The guiding principle of hormonal therapy of carcinoma of the breast is that both estrogens and androgens be reserved for patients whose disease is not amenable to surgical control. Androgen therapy may be expected to produce observable benefit in roughly 20 per cent of patients.

The observation that some women with carcinoma of the breast treated with androgens become polycythemic led to the use of these hormones to stimulate erythropoiesis in anemic patients with myeloid metaplasia and certain neoplastic diseases, such as multiple myeloma.[64, 65] Both in carcinoma of the breast and as an erythropoietic stimulant, androgens are used in doses significantly larger than physiologic, and their effects may not be apparent for 6 to 12 weeks.

The esters of testosterone are metabolized by the liver in a manner similar to that of the parent compound. The metabolic products appear in the urine. The esters are less polar than is testosterone itself and, when injected in oil, are absorbed more slowly and produce a more sustained effect. The halogenated testosterone derivatives are effectively absorbed from the gastrointestinal epithelium. Their mode of metabolism is poorly understood.

A number of androgenic preparations are available (Table 2–5 and Fig. 2–5). Among the most widely used are the ones given intramuscularly: testosterone propionate (Perandren, available in oil, 25 and 50 mg. per ml.); testosterone enanthate (Delatestryl, 200 mg. per ml.); and testosterone cypionate (Depo-testosterone, 50 to 200 mg. per ml.). These compounds are usually given 2 or 3 times weekly in single doses of 50 to 200 mg. per ml. and total weekly dosages of 200 to 1200 mg. Orally effective preparations such as fluoxymesterone (Halotestin, 2, 5, and 10 mg. tablets) are administered in divided doses of 10 to 40 mg. daily.

The most frequently encountered undesirable side effect of androgen therapy is virilization of female patients, a manifestation that is related to dosage and duration of therapy. Some new androgenic agents under study are reported to have less virilizing effect with the same antitumor properties. These new drugs are not generally available at present.

Androgens also frequently produce changes in libido and personality, induce fluid retention, and worsen symptoms of prostatic obstruction. The orally effective halogenated androgens can all produce cholestatic jaundice, which may necessitate withdrawal of the drug. Rarely androgens appear to cause exacerbation of the malignant process and, in patients with osteolytic lesions of breast cancer, may worsen hypercalcemia.

ADRENOCORTICOSTEROIDS. The pharmacology, principal therapeutic uses, and undesirable side effects of adrenocorticosteroids are so well known as to require little discussion here.[66] One of the major uses of these hormones in chemotherapy is in the treatment of malignant hematologic diseases, including acute lymphoblastic leukemia, chronic lymphocytic leukemia, lymphomas, and multiple myeloma. Adrenal hormones are used in these disorders as primary cytotoxic agents, as well as to control complications such as hemolytic anemia, thrombocytopenia, and hypercalcemia. The mechanism of their cytotoxic action is not understood, despite the voluminous literature. These hormones have an important place in the reduction of edema associated with therapy for spinal cord compression induced by leukemia or lymphoma. Adrenocorticosteroids may also have transient beneficial effects in a few nonhematologic malignancies, for example, carcinoma of the breast (Chap. 4), and metastatic carcinoma of the prostate (Chap. 3).

Several general principles govern the use of adrenocorticosteroids in malignant hematologic diseases. These compounds are usually used in very large doses for the minimal period of time necessary to achieve the desired clinical response, e.g., induction of a remission in acute lymphocytic leukemia or control of thrombocytopenia in chronic lymphocytic leukemia. The doses are then tapered to the minimal maintenance level, or withdrawn entirely in the case of acute lymphoblastic leukemia. It is generally wiser to start with a large dose and gradually reduce the level than to work slowly up to the maximal therapeutic dose. A preparation inducing minimal fluid retention, such as prednisone (oral) or prednisolone (intravenous), is generally used. The dosage varies, but is generally in the range of

40 to 120 mg. per day in adults, with a correspondingly reduced dosage in children. There is, at present, no evidence to suggest that an every-other-day schedule of steroid hormone administration is as effective as daily treatment for induction of remission in malignant hematologic diseases.

If adrenocorticosteroids are used for the appropriate periods of time indicated for malignant hematologic disease, long-term, undesirable side effects are rarely observed (e.g., osteoporosis, striae, purpura, truncal obesity). The short-term side effects do, however, frequently complicate the treatment of malignancy. These include diabetes mellitus, fluid and sodium retention, potassium loss, gastric irritation, and psychosis. Appropriate countermeasures should always be used in conjunction with adrenocorticosteroid therapy.

REFERENCES

1. Wheeler, G. P.: Studies related to the mechanisms of action of cytotoxic alkylating agents: A review. Cancer Res., 22:651–688, 1962.
2. Crathorn, A. R., and Roberts, J. J.: Mechanism of the cytotoxic action of alkylating agents in mammalian cells and evidence for the removal of alkylated groups from deoxyribonucleic acid. Nature, 211:150–153, 1966.
3. Little, J. B.: Cellular effects of ionizing radiation. New Eng. J. Med., 278:308, 1968.
4. Ochoa, M., Jr., and Hirschberg, E.: Alkylating agents. In Schnitzer, R. J., and Hawking, F. (Editors): Chemotherapy of Neoplastic Disease. New York, Academic Press, Inc., 1967, Vol. II, p. 1.
5. Calabresi, P., and Welch, A. D.: Chemotherapy of neoplastic diseases. Ann. Rev. Med., 13:147–202, 1962.
6. Godwin, H. A., Zimmerman, T. S., Kimball, H. R., Wolff, S. M., and Perry, S.: The effect of etiocholanolone on the entry of granulocytes into the peripheral blood. Blood, 31:461–470, 1968.
7. Foley, G. E., Friedman, O. M., and Drolet, B. P.: Studies on the mechanism of action of Cytoxan. Evidence of activation in vivo and in vitro. Cancer Res., 21:57–63, 1961.
8. Coggins, P. R., Ravdin, R. G., and Eisman, S. H.: Clinical evaluation of a new alkylating agent. Cancer, 13:1245, 1960.
9. Hall, T. C.: Pharmacologic studies of cyclophosphamide (NSC-26271) and its cogener phosphoramide mustard (NSC–69945). Cancer Chemother. Rep., 51:335–340, 1967.
10. Philips, F. S., Sternberg, S. S., Cronin, A. P., and Vidal, P. M.: Cyclophosphamide and urinary bladder toxicity. Cancer Res., 21:1577–1589, 1961.
11. Galton, D. A. G., Wiltshaw, E., Szur, L., and Dacie, J. V.: The use of chlorambucil and steroids in the treatment of chronic lymphocytic leukaemia. Brit. J. Haemat., 7:73–98, 1961.
12. Ezdinli, E. Z., and Stutzman, L.: Chlorambucil therapy for lymphomas and chronic lymphocytic leukemia. J.A.M.A., 191:444–450, 1965.
13. Freckman, H. A., Fry, H. L., Mendez, F. L., and Maurer, E. R.: Chlorambucil-prednisone therapy for disseminated breast carcinoma. J.A.M.A., 189:23, 1964.
14. Vaitkevicius, F. K., Talley, R. W., Brennan, M. J., and Kelly, J. E.: Chemotherapy of advanced ovarian cancer. J. Michigan Med. Soc., 60:492, 1961.
15. White, F. R.: New agent data summaries. Sarcolysin and related compounds. Cancer Chemother. Rep. 6:61, 1960.
16. Waldenström, J.: Melphalan therapy in myelomatosis. Brit. Med. J., 1:859–865, 1964.
17. Bergsagel, D. E., Migliore, P. J., and Griffith, K. M.: Myeloma proteins and the clinical response to melphalan therapy. Science, 148:376, 1965.

18. Vodopick, H. A., Hamilton, H. E., Jackson, H. B., Peng, C. T., and Sheets, R. F.: Studies on the fate of tritiated busulfan in man. J. Clin. Invest., 42:989, 1963.

19. Nadkarni, M. V., Trams, E. G., and Smith, P. K.: Preliminary studies on the distribution and fate of TEM, TEPA, and Myleran in the human. Cancer Res., 19:713, 1959.

20. Kyle, R. A., Schwartz, R. S., Oliner, H. L., and Dameshek, W.: A syndrome resembling adrenal cortical insufficiency associated with long term busulfan (Myleran) therapy. Blood, 18:497–510, 1961.

21. Kyle, R. A., and Dameshek, W.: Porphyria cutanea tarda associated with chronic granulocytic leukemia treated with busulfan (Myleran). Blood, 23:776–785, 1964.

22. Leake, E., Smith, W. G., and Woodliff, H. J.: Diffuse interstitial pulmonary fibrosis after busulphan therapy. Lancet, ii:432–434, 1963.

23. Farber, S., Diamond, L. K., Mercer, R. D., Sylvester, R. F., Jr., and Wolff, J. A.: Temporary remission in acute leukemia in children produced by folic acid antagonist, 4-aminopteroyl-glutamic acid (aminopterin). New Eng. J. Med., 238:787, 1948.

24. Friedkin, M.: Enzymatic aspects of folic acid. Ann. Rev. Biochem., 32:185, 1963.

25. Bertino, J. R., Booth, B. A., Bieber, A. L., Cashmore, A., and Sartorelli, A. C.: Studies on the inhibition of dihydrofolate reductase by the folate antagonists. J. Biol. Chem., 239:479–485, 1964.

26. Condit, P. T., Chanes, R. E., and Joel, W.: Renal toxicity of methotrexate. Cancer, 23:126, 1969.

27. Coe, R. A., and Bull, F. E.: Cirrhosis associated with methotrexate treatment of psoriasis. J.A.M.A., 206:1515–1520, 1968.

28. Bertino, J. R., Donohue, D. M., Simmons, B., Gabrio, B. W., Silber, R., and Huennekens, F. M.: The "induction" of dihydrofolic reductase activity in leukocytes and erythrocytes of patients treated with amethopterin. J. Clin. Invest., 42:466, 1963.

29. Fischer, G. A., Bertino, J. R., Calabresi, P., Clement, D. H., Zanes, R. P., Lyman, M. S., Burchenal, J. H., and Welch, A. D.: Uptake of tritium-labeled methotrexate by human leukemic leukocytes. Blood, 22:819–820, 1963.

30. Djerassi, I.: Methotrexate infusions and intensive supportive care in the management of children with acute lymphocytic leukemia: Follow-up report. Cancer Res., 27:2561–2564, 1967.

31. Berlin, N. I., Rall, D., Mead, J. A. R., Freireich, E. J., Van Scott, E., Hertz, R., and Lipsett, M. B.: Folic acid antagonists. Effects on the cell and the patient. Combined clinical staff conference at the National Institutes of Health. Ann. Intern. Med., 59:931–956, 1963.

32. Bertino, J. R., and Johns, D. G.: Folate antagonists. Ann. Rev. Med., 18:27–34, 1967.

33. Elion, G. B., Burge, E., and Hitchings, G. H.: Studies on condensed pyrimidine systems. IX. The synthesis of some 6-substituted purines. J. Amer. Chem. Soc., 74:411, 1952.

34. Elion, G. B., Callahan, S., Rundles, R. W., and Hitchings, G. H.: Relationship between metabolic fates and antitumor activities of thiopurines. Cancer Res., 23:1207–1217, 1963.

35. Hitchings, G. H., and Elion, G. B.: Mechanism of action of purine and pyrimidine analogs. In Brodsky, I., Kahn, S. B., and Moyer, J. H. (Editors): Cancer Chemotherapy. New York, Grune & Stratton, Inc., 1967, p. 26.

36. Elion, G. B.: Biochemistry and pharmacology of purine analogues. Fed. Proc., 26:898–904, 1967.

37. Loo, T. L., Luce, J. K., Sullivan, M. P., and Frei, E., III: Clinical pharmacologic observations on 6-mercaptopurine and 6-methylthiopurine ribonucleoside. Clin. Pharm. Therap., 9:180–194, 1968.

38. Einhorn, M., and Davidsohn, I.: Hepatotoxicity of mercaptopurine. J.A.M.A., 188:802–806, 1964.

39. Shorey, J., Schenker, S., Suki, W. N., and Combes, B.: Hepatotoxicity of mercaptopurine. Arch. Intern. Med., 122:54, 1968.

40. Heidelberger, C., and Ansfield, F. J.: Experimental and clinical use of fluorinated pyrimidines in cancer chemotherapy. Cancer Res., 23:1226–1243, 1963.

41. Reyes, P., and Heidelberger, C.: Fluorinated purines. XXVI. Mammalian thymidylate synthetase: Its mechanism of action and inhibition by fluorinated nucleotides. Mol. Pharmacol., 1:14–30, 1965.
42. Clarkson, B., O'Connor, A., Winston, L., and Hutchison, D.: The physiologic disposition of 5-fluorouracil and 5-fluoro-2'-deoxyuridine in man. Clin. Pharm. Therap., 5:581–610, 1964.
42a. Jacobs, E. M., Luce, J. K., and Wood, D. A.: Treatment of cancer with weekly intravenous 5-fluorouracil. Cancer, 22:1233–1238, 1968.
43. Ansfield, F. J., Schroeder, J. M., and Curreri, A. R.: Five years' clinical experience with 5-fluorouracil. J.A.M.A., 181:295–299, 1962.
44. Chu, M. Y., and Fischer, G. A.: A proposed mechanism of action of 1-β-D-arabinofuranosyl-cytosine as an inhibitor of the growth of leukemic cells. Biochem. Pharmacol., 11:423–430, 1962.
45. Howard, J. P., Albo, V., and Newton, W. A.: Cytosine arabinoside. Results of a cooperative study in acute childhood leukemia. Cancer, 21:341, 1968.
46. Talley, R. W., O'Bryan, R. M., Tucker, W. G., and Loo, R. V.: Clinical pharmacology and human antitumor activity of cytosine arabinoside. Cancer, 20:809, 1967.
47. Creasey, W. A., Papac, R. J., Markiw, M. E., Calabresi, P., and Welch, A. D.: Biochemical and pharmacological studies with 1-β-D-arabinofuranosylcytosine in man. Biochem. Pharm., 15:1417–1428, 1966.
48. Burke, P. J., Serpick, A. A., Carbone, P. P., and Tarr, N.: A clinical evaluation of dose and schedule of administration of cytosine arabinoside (NSC 63878). Cancer Res., 28:274–279, 1968.
49. Waksman, S. A., and Woodruff, H. B.: Bacteriostatic and bactericidal substances produced by a soil actinomyces. Proc. Soc. Exp. Biol. Med., 45:609, 1940.
50. Reich, E.: Biochemistry of actinomycins. Cancer Res., 23:1428–1441, 1963.
51. Goldstein, M. N., Hamm, K., and Amrod, E.: Incorporation of tritiated actinomycin-D into drug-sensitive and drug-resistant HeLa cells. Science, 151:1555–1556, 1966.
52. Brown, J. H., and Kennedy, B. J.: Mithramycin in the treatment of disseminated testicular neoplasms. New Eng. J. Med., 272:111, 1965.
53. Tan, C., Tasaka, H., Yu, K.-P., Murphy, M. L., and Karnofsky, D. A.: Daunomycin, an antitumor antibiotic, in the treatment of neoplastic disease. Clinical evaluation with special reference to childhood leukemia. Cancer, 20:333–353, 1967.
54. Johnson, I. S., Armstrong, J. G., Gorman, M., and Burnett, J. P.: The vinca alkaloids: A new class of oncolytic agents. Cancer Res., 23:1390–1427, 1963.
55. Armstrong, J. G.: The mechanism of action of the vinca alkaloids. In Brodsky, I., Kahn, S. B., and Moyer, J. H. (Editors): Cancer Chemotherapy. New York, Grune & Stratton, Inc., 1967, p. 37.
56. Creasey, W. A.: Modifications in biochemical pathways produced by the vinca alkaloids. Cancer Chemother. Rep., 52:501–507, 1968.
57. Cline, M. J.: Effect of vincristine on synthesis of ribonucleic acid and protein in leukaemic leucocytes. Brit. J. Haemat., 14:21–29, 1968.
58. Slater, L. M., Wainer, R. A., and Serpick, A. A.: Vincristine neurotoxicity with hyponatremia. Cancer, 23:122, 1969.
59. Huggins, C., Stevens, R. E., Jr., and Hodges, C. V.: Studies on prostatic cancer: effects of castration on advanced carcinoma of prostate gland. Arch. Surg., 43:209, 1941.
60. Haddow, A., Watkinson, J. M., and Paterson, E.: Influence of synthetic oestrogens upon advanced malignant disease. Brit. Med., J., 2:393, 1944.
61. Wade, R.: Hormones. In Schnitzer, R. J., and Hawkins, F. (Editors): Experimental Chemotherapy. New York, Academic Press, Inc., 1967, Vol. V, Part II, p. 133.
62. Dodds, E. C., Golberg, L., Lawson, W., and Robinson, R.: Oestrogenic activity of alkylated stilboestrols. Nature, 142:34, 1938.
63. Loeser, A. A.: Mammary carcinoma: response to implantation of male hormone and progesterone. Lancet, ii:698, 1941.
64. Gardner, F. H., and Nathan, D. G.: Androgens and erythropoiesis: Further evaluation of testosterone treatment of myelofibrosis. New Eng. J. Med., 274:420, 1966.

65. Cline, M. J., and Berlin, N. I.: Studies of the anemia of multiple myeloma. Amer. J. Med., 33:510–525, 1962.
66. Travis, R. H., and Sayers, G.: Adrenocorticotropic hormone; adrenocortical steroids and their synthetic analogs. In Goodman, L. S., and Gilman, A. (Editors): The Pharmacological Basis of Therapeutics. Ed. 3. New York, The Macmillan Company, 1965, p. 1608.
67. Bollag, W.: Suppression of the immunological reaction by methylhydrazines, a new class of antitumor agents. Experientia, 19:304, 1963.
68. Chaube, S., and Murphy, M. L.: Fetal malformations produced in rats by N-isopropyl-α-(2-methylhydrazino)-p-toluamide HCl (procarbazine). Teratology, 2:23, 1969.
69. Kelly, M. G., O'Gara, R. W., Godekar, K., Yancey, S. T., and Oliverio, V. T.: Carcinogenic activity of a new antitumor agent, N-isopropyl-α-(2-methylhydrazino)-p-hydrochloride (NSC–77213). Cancer Chemother. Rep., 39:77, 1964.
70. Rutishauser, A., and Bollag, W.: Cytological investigations with a new class of cytotoxic agents: Methylhydrazine derivatives. Experientia, 19:131, 1963.
71. Bollag, W., and Grunberg, E.: Tumor inhibitory effects of a new class of cytotoxic agents: Methylhydrazine derivatives. Experientia, 19:130, 1963.
72. Brunner, K. W., and Young, C. W.: A methylhydrazine derivative in Hodgkin's disease and other malignant neoplasms. Therapeutic and toxic effects studied in 51 patients. Ann. Intern. Med., 63:69–86, 1965.

Additional Recent Bibliography Not Cited in Text

73. Rutman, R. J., Chun, E. H. L., and Jones, J.: Observations on the mechanism of the alkylation reaction between nitrogen mustard and DNA. Biochim. Biophys. Acta, 174:663–673, 1969.
74. Wolpert, M. K., and Ruddon, R. W.: A study on the mechanism of resistance to nitrogen mustard (HN_2) in Ehrlich ascites tumor cells: Comparison of uptake of HN_2-^{14}C into sensitive and resistant cells. Cancer Res., 29:873–879, 1969.
75. Elion, G. B.: Actions of purine analogs: Enzyme specificity studies as a basis for interpretation and design. Cancer Res., 29:2448–2453, 1969.
76. Kessel, D., Hall, T. C., and Rosenthal, D.: Uptake and phosphorylation of cytosine arabinoside by normal and leukemic human blood cells in vitro. Cancer Res., 29:459–463, 1969.
77. Karon, M., and Shirakawa, S.: The locus of action of 1-β-D-Arabinofuranosylcytosine in the cell cycle. Cancer Res., 29:687–696, 1969.
78. Northrop, G., Taylor, S. G., III, and Northrop, R. L.: Biochemical effects of mithramycin on cultured cells. Cancer Res., 29:1916–1919, 1969.
79. Epstein, E. H., Jr., and Lutzner, M. A.: Folliculitis induced by actinomycin-D. New Eng. J. Med., 281:1094, 1969.
80. Creasey, W. A.: Biochemical effects of the vinca alkaloids. IV. Studies with vinleurosine. Biochem. Pharmacol., 18:227–232, 1969.
81. Bensch, K. G., Marantz, R., Wisniewski, H., and Shelanski, M.: Induction in vitro of microtubular crystals by vinca alkaloids. Science, 165:495–496, 1969.
82. Dowling, M. D., Jr., Krakoff, I. H., and Karnofsky, D. A.: Mechanism of action of anticancer drugs. In Cole, W. H. (Editor): Chemotherapy of Cancer. Philadelphia, Lea & Febiger, 1970.

CHAPTER 3

GENITOURINARY MALIGNANCY

CARCINOMA OF THE PROSTATE

Prostatic cancer is considered to be the most common form of cancer in men over 50 years of age. It is an insidious disease. The early lesion is usually so far from the urethra that many patients do not develop urinary symptoms until malignancy has progressed beyond the surgically curable stage; over 90 per cent of patients have nonresectable disease at the time of diagnosis.

The usual sequence of therapeutic procedures for metastatic carcinoma of the prostate is schematized in Figure 3–1. The pioneering studies of Huggins[1] and his collaborators in the early 1940's led to the introduction of androgen-control therapy for carcinoma of the prostate. In a large majority of affected patients, prostatic tumors and their metastases are hormone sensitive and respond to endocrine therapy. In metastatic disease, surgical eradication of the primary neoplasm is not indicated unless it is large and producing local symptoms. Orchiectomy is the initial treatment in disseminated disease and can be expected to produce remissions that may last for several years in a majority of the patients. There is no evidence that orchiectomy combined with estrogen therapy is superior to orchiectomy alone.

Endocrine therapy may be successful in the small fraction of patients who do not respond to orchiectomy and in those who relapse after an initial response.[1] Androgen control is generally achieved within a few weeks by conventional doses of estrogen, which suppress the production of testosterone by the testes and of luteinizing hormone

42

by the pituitary.[2] Diethylstilbestrol is an inexpensive and effective synthetic estrogen used for this purpose. It is often given initially in a dosage of 3 to 5 mg. per day orally and subsequently reduced to 1 to 3 mg. per day for maintenance of remission. Response to therapy is usually heralded by relief of pain and improvement of performance status and appetite. Subjective improvement is usually associated with objective tumor regression and a fall in the serum acid phosphatase. The most frequent early side effect of diethylstilbestrol therapy is nausea, which, however, usually disappears with continued therapy. Fluid retention is a common complication; carcinoma of the male breast is a very rare complication.

In the case of patients whose disease has relapsed after orchiectomy and subsequent estrogen treatment, adrenocorticosteroids should be tried. Remissions induced by these agents are usually of shorter duration than those produced by orchiectomy and estrogens. Prednisone in a dosage of 30 to 60 mg. per day usually suffices to induce a response. Thereafter, the dosage is reduced to the minimal level necessary for maintaining remission.

Patients who fail to respond to adrenal steroids may be candidates for adrenalectomy or for chemotherapy (alkylating agents or 5-FU). There has been relatively little experience with cytotoxic agents in treating this disease and there are, as yet, no definitive guidelines for therapy. Busulfan appears to be ineffective.[3] The physicians of the U.S. Veterans Administration hospitals have had considerable experience in the treatment of this disease and have accumulated much of the clinically useful data.[4]

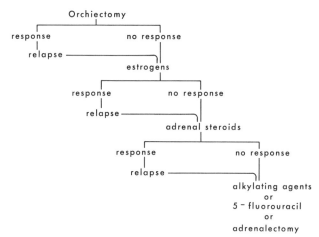

Figure 3–1   Usual sequence of therapy in patients with metastatic carcinoma of the prostate.

ENDOMETRIAL CARCINOMA OF THE CORPUS UTERI

Patients with adenocarcinoma of the endometrium are character-ized by a high frequency of sterility and an unusual frequency of metrorrhagia during the menopause. Diabetes mellitus and hyperten-sion are said to be frequently associated diseases; however, the evi-dence for this is not convincing.

The initial treatment of early stages of carcinoma of the corpus uteri is surgery, perhaps in combination with radiation therapy. Ap-proximately two-thirds of the patients with this disease receive initial treatment when the malignancy is clinically localized in the uterus, and about 70 per cent of them can anticipate survival of at least five years. For excellent reviews of the staging and primary treatment of this malignancy, the reader is referred to the works of Barber and Brunschweig[5] and of Truskett and Constable.[6]

In stage III and IV disease, when the tumor has extended beyond the confines of the uterus, the physician has a choice of more exten-sive surgery such as pelvic exenteration, more extensive radiation therapy, or chemotherapy. There is a limited place for pelvic exenter-ation in the treatment of recurrent endometrial carcinoma, but the patients must be carefully selected.[5] In advanced disease no longer amenable to surgical or radiotherapeutic attack, chemotherapy must be considered.

Kelly and Baker[7, 8] were among the first to demonstrate the effectiveness of progestational agents in this disorder. Between 20 and 50 per cent of patients show an objective response to large doses of progestins. The optimal dose of hydroxyprogesterone caproate (Dela-lutin) recommended by Kistner et al.[9] is 3 to 5 gm. intramuscularly, weekly for at least 6 weeks. If remission occurs, therapy is continued at maintenance dose levels. Another progestational agent, medroxy-progesterone acetate (Depo-Provera), is given for 6 weeks in doses of at least 3 gm. per week. Maintenance therapy of 400 to 500 mg. daily by mouth is continued thereafter if remission is induced.

Pulmonary and osseous lesions of metastatic endometrial carcin-oma respond to progestational agents more frequently than do visceral lesions.[9] Patients who respond to treatment survive longer (21.6 months after initiation of therapy) than those who do not respond (7.8 months).[9]

In general, the response of patients with stage III and IV disease to treatment with cytotoxic agents has been unsatisfactory. Only rare-ly do endometrial tumors show objective response to treatment with conventional doses of alkylating agents or methotrexate.

Gynecologic sarcomas or so-called "pelvic sarcomas" are rare, and no extensive chemotherapeutic experience has accumulated. Mal-kasian[10] and his colleagues treated patients with such neoplasms with either actinomycin-D plus radiation or with 5-FU; they observed objective tumor responses lasting 3 to 10 months in 9 of 19 treated patients. Leiomyosarcomas may be more responsive than other gynecologic sarcomas.

OVARIAN CARCINOMA

Survival data for 1722 patients with carcinoma of the ovary of various histologic types have been compiled by Maus et al.[11] Surgery and radiation therapy are the principal modalities of treatment for ovarian carcinoma of all types, including serous and mucinous cystadenocarcinoma, endometrioid carcinoma, tumors of germ-cell origin, and the rare hormone-producing and unclassified tumors.

In extensive disease no longer amenable to surgery and radiation therapy, chemotherapeutic agents must be considered. Cystadenocarcinoma is the commonest malignant tumor of the ovary. After it had been recognized that this tumor was frequently sensitive to alkylating agents, a great variety of alkylators were tried.[12] All of them seemed to produce comparable rates of objective tumor regression, roughly 30 to 50 per cent. Consequently, the choice of agent is dictated by other considerations, such as route of administration, rapidity of action, vesicant effect, and cost.[13] It is likely that alkylators do not significantly prolong survival in patients with disseminated carcinoma of the ovary.[14] There is no question, however, that they can reduce morbidity in patients with responsive tumors.

Intravenous administration of nitrogen mustard (0.2 to 0.4 mg. per kg.) or cyclophosphamide (15 to 30 mg. per kg. in divided doses) can be used when a rapid effect is desired. Oral administration of chlorambucil, 2 to 6 mg. per day,[15] or cyclophosphamide, 75 to 150 mg. per day,[16] is equally effective but usually slower in the induction of regression. Oral administration of melphalan is also effective,[17] but in my experience is a more difficult alkylating agent to use.

Thiotepa in a single dose of 0.04 to 0.8 mg. per kg. may be given intrapleurally or intra-abdominally in cases of intractable pleural effusion or ascites. This drug's vesicating action is less severe than that of nitrogen mustard and it is preferable for intra-abdominal use. Systemic effects are often observed after intracavitary use of either this alkylating agent or nitrogen mustard, and the white blood cell and platelet counts may fall within 7 to 12 days.

The experience with agents other than alkylating agents in the treatment of carcinoma of the ovary is meager and difficult to evaluate. 5-FU and methotrexate in combination with alkylating agents,[18] and actinomycin-D,[19] have all been tried with occasional success. Such treatment should be reserved for problem cases, when radiation therapy can no longer be used and when alkylating agents are ineffective. Insufficient data are available at present to evaluate concurrent use of radiation therapy and either alkylating agents or other cytotoxic agents.

ILLUSTRATIVE CASE HISTORY: CARCINOMA OF THE OVARY

A 48-year-old woman noted the gradual onset of increased abdominal girth and constipation in *September 1965*; 3 months later she experienced an episode of severe abdominal distention associated with colic pain and was referred by her physician to the University of California Hospitals, San Francisco.

In *February 1966*, pelvic examination showed that the uterus was displaced anteriorly by a hard irregular mass, which filled the cul de sac and extended laterally to the pelvic walls. Shortly thereafter surgery was performed and revealed an ovarian tumor (a papillary cystadenocarcinoma, 15 cm. in diameter) filling the right half of the pelvis. The tumor had broken through its capsule, and there were numerous small implants in the omentum and on the surface of the liver and the peritoneum. The sigmoid colon was compressed but not invaded by the tumor. A major portion of the mass was removed and a bilateral salpingo-oophorectomy was performed. A radiation therapist was present during the surgical procedures.

Eleven days postoperatively, radiation therapy was begun. After only two weeks of therapy (1550 rads, midplane pelvis) the patient was hospitalized because of peritonitis and a pelvic abscess, which were treated with antibiotics.

The decision was then made to discontinue radiation therapy and to begin chemotherapy with chlorambucil, 4 to 6 mg. per day, given orally. At this time (*April 1966*) the patient had bilateral pleural effusions, ascites, hepatomegaly, and a suprapubic mass (6 by 6 cm.). She complained of pain at the left costovertebral angle; this was attributed to a metastatic lesion. The dose of chlorambucil was adjusted to keep the white blood count above 4000 per cu. mm. Within 8 weeks after the beginning of therapy the effusions had disappeared, and the liver and suprapubic mass were no longer palpable. The patient had gained 11 pounds and had returned to work. On *June 20, 1966*, chlorambucil therapy was stopped because of the development of leukopenia.

The patient was temporarily lost to follow-up, but returned early in *September 1966* with recurrent abdominal pain and constipation. A large mass involving the entire posterior pelvis was palpated and thought to be producing a partial obstruction of the sigmoid. A tender right suprapubic mass (10 by 10 cm.) was also palpated. Bone marrow aspiration revealed hypoplastic marrow and metastatic carcinoma. Chlorambucil was resumed at a dose of 4 mg. per day, and again the patient's condition improved strikingly with reduction in the size of both masses and return of the bone marrow to normal.

The patient was asymptomatic from *October 1966* to *November 1967*. Chlorambucil was continued at various doses until *November 1967*, when the patient returned to the hospital because of recurrent pleural effusion containing malignant cells. Thiotepa, 0.6 mg. per kg., was instilled intrapleurally after removal of 1500 ml. of blood-containing fluid. Effusions were controlled by this measure. However, the patient's condition slowly deteriorated until *February 1968*, when in her home she suddenly bled massively from the tumor involving the cecum. Therapeutic efforts were unsuccessful, and the patient died.

COMMENT: This patient with inoperable metastatic carcinoma of the ovary clearly benefited from therapy with an alkylating agent which was administered for a period of 16 months. Chlorambucil produced an objective response (a reduction in accumulated fluid and size of masses), as well as subjective improvement. The level of the white blood cell count was used as a guide to the dosage of chlorambucil. Recurrent malignant pleural effusions developed while the patient was receiving chlorambucil. These effusions responded to intrapleural administration of Thiotepa.

If the patient had survived longer, she would have been placed on an experimental protocol and treated with 5-fluorouracil, since it was apparent that alkylating agents were no longer effective in the control of her disease.

TROPHOBLASTIC TUMORS OF THE UTERUS

Trophoblastic tumors, despite their rarity, are of special interest to the chemotherapist, representing one of the two malignancies curable by chemical agents alone. The cure rate achieved with chemotherapeutic management of trophoblastic tumors approaches 90 per cent. This fact is not yet universally appreciated, with the consequence that surgery and radiation therapy are sometimes still employed as primary treatment for metastatic disease. However, the cure rate with surgery and radiation therapy is considerably lower than with chemotherapy.

The explanation of the curability of trophoblastic tumors by chemical agents is not entirely clear. Trophoblastic tissue is a product of conception, a homotransplant, genetically a back-cross to the female. It has been suggested that these tumors contain histocompatibility loci not present in the host, with the consequence that the host's immunologic defenses are mobilized against the malignant tissue.[20] So far, specific antibodies have not been discovered.

This disease can progress rapidly. Once the diagnosis is established, it is mandatory that chemotherapy be started as soon as possible. The shorter the duration of disease before chemotherapy, the greater the likelihood of complete remission.[21] If treatment is delayed as much as 4 to 6 months after symptoms develop, the prognosis is poor.

The pathologic classification of trophoblastic malignancy is as follows:[22]

Hydatidiform mole: classified as apparently benign, potentially malignant, and apparently malignant.

Chorioadenoma destruens (invasive mole): a malignant mole with local invasion of the myometrium or its vessels with one or more villi, or with distant metastases.

Choriocarcinoma: malignant trophoblastic tissue composed of chorionic cells, without evidence of villus formation, invading the myometrium and its vessels, and frequently metastatic.

Choriocarcinoma and chorioadenoma destruens have the same prognosis and clinically may be regarded as the same disease. Slightly more than 50 per cent of the cases of choriocarcinoma follow a hydatidiform mole, 25 per cent follow an abortion, and roughly 20 per cent are preceded by an apparently normal pregnancy. The remaining 2 or 3 per cent follow an ectopic pregnancy. When choriocarcinoma is diagnosed, the course of action is clear. A more difficult problem for the clinician may be the management of the patient who has passed a hydatidiform mole. Such moles occur approximately once in 2000 pregnancies among occidental patients and at roughly 10 times that frequency in certain oriental populations. Between 2 and 5 per cent of moles are followed by malignant trophoblastic disease.

Trophoblastic tumors are the only neoplasms that may be treated without histopathologic verification of malignancy. If the clinical picture is sufficiently suspicious and the chorionic gonadotropin titer is very high, the physician may be justified in beginning chemotherapy even if uterine curettage has not yielded malignant tissue. Overambitious attempts at obtaining tissue from other sites may result in unnecessary delays and in some cases expose the patient to a high operative risk.

When does one decide that a mole is malignant, or that choriocarcinoma is present in the absence of a clearly positive histologic examination? The guidelines are as follows: After passage of a mole, dilatation and curettage should be performed promptly. The chorionic gonadotropin titer should be followed carefully for at least 8 weeks. If the titer remains elevated and shows no evidence of returning to a baseline, the patient is regarded as having malignant trophoblastic disease.[23, 24] A high titer indicates that the tumor contains trophoblastic tissue and that the cells are still active endocrinologically, secreting chorionic gonadotropin—thus serving as an endocrine marker indicating their presence in the body.

The sequence of therapy used in choriocarcinoma is outlined in Figure 3-2. There is no indication for hysterectomy in the treatment of metastatic disease unless uterine hemorrhage is uncontrollable. Hysterectomy does not improve the chances for survival and, indeed,

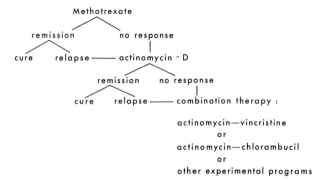

Figure 3–2   Usual sequence of chemotherapy in patients with choriocarcinoma.

may possibly prejudice the results of chemotherapy.[25] A patient cured of a trophoblastic tumor with an intact uterus may subsequently bear children.

The initial therapy of choice is the antifolic acid compound, methotrexate, given intermittently in large doses; for example, 15 to 25 mg. intravenously daily for 4 or 5 days.[24, 26, 27] Such a course may be repeated at intervals of 2 or 4 weeks, as permitted by toxicity. Undesirable side effects are often significant at these high dose levels, and include myelosuppression with leukopenia and thrombocytopenia and hepatic, renal, and central nervous system toxicity. Toxicity usually regresses completely with discontinuance of the drug. If remission occurs, treatment should be continued for 4 to 6 months after all evidence of disease is gone. The patient should be given periodic physical examinations and appropriate radiologic examinations for renal and pulmonary involvement, and chorionic gonadotropin titers should be determined at frequent intervals. A sensitive test for chorionic gonadotropin should be used, such as the modified Aschheim-Zondek test, or preferably an immunologic assay should be used in following the patient.[25] Treatment should be continued until the titer falls below 200 International Units (IU) in 24 hours. Titers should be determined at monthly intervals for at least 2 years.

Fifty to 75 per cent of the patients can expect a remission when treated with methotrexate.[29] Drug resistance develops in roughly half the patients in whom methotrexate is initially effective. Remissions with methotrexate are related to the duration of the disease before therapy, to the extent of the disease at the time of therapy, and to the chorionic gonadotropin titer. Only 30 per cent of patients with titers greater than 1,000,000 IU obtain a remission, whereas 75 per cent of those with lower titers respond.

If the patient develops resistance to methotrexate or does not respond to this drug, actinomycin-D should be used.[30] Actinomycin-D is given intravenously either once weekly in a dose of 2 to 2.5 mg.

in 250 ml. of saline or in daily doses of 0.5 gm. for 5 days. Such courses may be repeated as toxicity permits.

A patient whose tumor does not respond to either methotrexate or actinomycin-D may respond to vincristine, 0.01 to 0.02 mg. per kg. once weekly, or chlorambucil, 8 mg. per day orally, may be added. If this program fails, additional therapy with 6-mercaptopurine[31] or vinblastine[32] should be considered.

In summary, the important points in the management of this potentially curable disease are: early institution of methotrexate therapy; sequential use of other drugs if the response to methotrexate is suboptimal; continuation of therapy for 4 to 6 months after all evidence of disease has disappeared; and follow-up with chorionic gonadotropin titer determinations and appropriate roentgenographic studies. Pregnancy should be delayed for at least 2 years after treatment is stopped in order that the chorionic gonadotropin titer can be used as a valid index of the activity of disease. The sequence of therapy in a patient with choriocarcinoma and the results that can be achieved are illustrated in Figures 3–3 and 3–4. For an excellent review of this complex subject, the reader is referred to the recent report of Johnson and colleagues.[27]

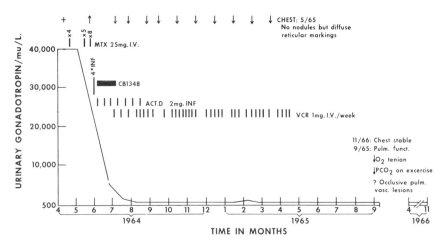

Figure 3-3 Therapy (methotrexate followed by chlorambucil and actinomycin D) and the hormonal response in a patient with metastatic choriocarcinoma. (From Johnson, F. D., Jacobs, E. M., and Silliphant, W. M.: Trophoblastic tumors of the uterus. Problems of methotrexate therapy. California Med., *108*:1–13, 1968. Reprinted by permission of the author and publisher.)

A

B

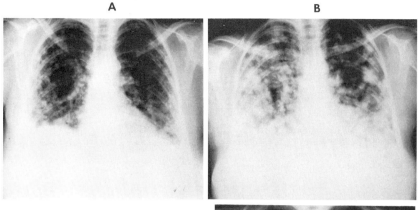

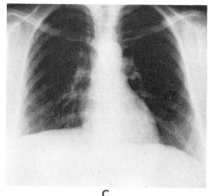

Figure 3-4 Same patient with metastatic choriocarcinoma (cf. Fig. 3-3). Serial chest roentgenograms during the course of therapy. (From Johnson, F. D., Jacobs, E. M., and Silliphant, W. M.: Trophoblastic tumors of the uterus. Problems of methotrexate therapy. California Med., *108*:1-13, 1968. Reprinted by permission of the author and publisher.)

C

ILLUSTRATIVE CASE HISTORY: CHORIOCARCINOMA

A 43-year-old Philippine woman who came to the United States from Manila in 1965 was thought to be in good health, except for an intermittent cough. In *June 1967*, dilatation and curettage were performed following passage of a hydatidiform mole. Examination of the histologic sections revealed atypical trophoblastic proliferation, but no myometrium was included in the sections and the presence or absence of myometrial invasion could not be ascertained. Chorionic gonadotropin titers were not obtained.

In *November 1968*, the patient developed a recurrent cough; other symptoms were night sweats and weight loss. In *June and July 1969*, she was seen at the general hospital in the county of her residence, where she was evaluated for tuberculosis. A radio-opaque lesion was found in the right upper lung and a strongly positive reaction to PPD was noted. The patient became disgruntled with her medical care and left the hospital before treatment was started. One week later, in late *July 1969*, she was admitted to the University of California Hospitals, San Francisco. At that time she appeared chronically ill and wasted. She was febrile (39° C.) and had a productive cough. Chest roentgenograms showed diffuse "fibronodular disease" bilaterally (Fig. 3-5). Urinary chorionic gonadotropin titers were positive (800,000 IU per liter). The possibility of pregnancy as a cause of the elevated titer was excluded by pelvic examination. The patient was considered to be too ill to

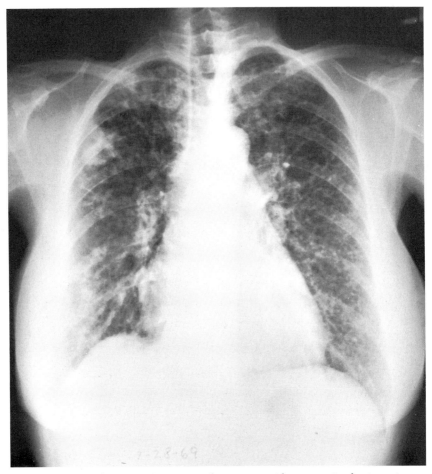

Figure 3-5   Chest roentgenogram of a patient with metastatic choriocarcinoma before therapy *(July 23, 1969).* See case history.

undergo a lung biopsy. Appropriate cultures were obtained for tuberculosis and fungal disease. (These later proved to be negative.)

Methotrexate therapy was started after a presumptive diagnosis of choriocarcinoma was made, without biopsy. Methotrexate was given intravenously, 15 mg. on each of 4 successive days. (Because tuberculosis could not be excluded at the time, antituberculosis therapy was begun simultaneously.) Within two weeks after beginning methotrexate treatment the patient appeared improved, and a second course of therapy was given. A total of four courses of methotrexate (40 to 60 mg. each) were given over a 6-week period, and the patient was discharged from the hospital. At that time urinary chorionic gonadotropin titers were negative (less than 800 IU per liter).

Over the subsequent two months the patient felt well and gained weight. The cough and fever disappeared, and the pulmonary lesions appeared improved on chest roentgenograms (Fig. 3–6).

Early in *October 1969*, an additional course of methotrexate was begun. Chorionic gonadotropin titers were still negative as of February 1970.

COMMENT: This patient should have been evaluated for choriocarcinoma very soon after passage of a hydatidiform mole because of the relatively high incidence of choriocarcinoma among women in the Philippines and the high incidence of choriocarcinoma preceded by a hydatidiform mole. Unfortunately, this diagnosis was not suspected until the patient developed severe pulmonary symptoms almost two years later. The diagnosis of choriocarcinoma was then made on the basis of her history, the pulmonary lesion, and a chorionic gonadotropin titer that was very high in the absence of pregnancy. Chemotherapy for choriocarcinoma was begun without benefit of a biopsy and a histopathologic diagnosis because of the high risk of a biopsy procedure in a critically ill woman with impaired ventilation. Methotrexate induced a dramatic clinical response, objectively and symptomatically. The pulmonary lesion improved, the chorionic gonadotropin titer was reduced, and the patient's symptoms disappeared.

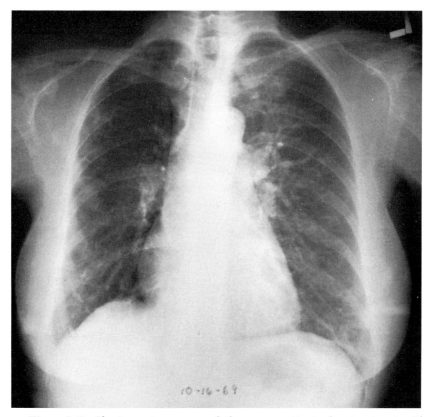

Figure 3–6 Chest roentgenogram of the same patient after treatment with methotrexate *(October 16, 1969)*. See case history.

TESTICULAR NEOPLASMS

The chemotherapist's zeal in attacking testicular neoplasms is not a reflection of their frequency, since these neoplasms constitute slightly less than 10 per cent of all malignant neoplasms of the male genitourinary tract. Testicular carcinoma frequently occurs in the young. The patient's physical condition may be good and he may be asymptomatic, but metastatic disease—often pulmonary—may have developed by the time of diagnosis. It is rewarding, if rare, to treat a young patient so that he is clinically free of his disease for several years and may have a chance of surviving his normal lifespan.

Testicular neoplasms include malignancies of germinal cell origin, gonadostromal neoplasms, the rare Sertoli cell tumor, androblastoma, and interstitial cell testicular tumor. In addition, there are a number of tumors that originate in supportive and paratesticular tissues. Practically all primary malignant tumors of the testis are of germinal cell origin, and this chapter is confined to these tumors. Germinal cell tumors predominate during the early decades of life. Their frequency decreases markedly after the sixth decade, when tumors of paratesticular origin account for roughly 75 per cent of testicular tumors.[33] Lymphomas account for over 40 per cent of testicular neoplasms after the age of 60. The approach to therapy of testicular lymphomas is the same as that of lymphomas originating in other sites, and is discussed elsewhere (cf. Chap. 12).

Testicular Tumors of Germinal Cell Origin

The histopathologic classification of germinal cell testicular tumors is important with respect to both prognosis and choice of initial therapy. The classification of Dixon and Moore[34] and the approximate relative frequency of each type of tumor in the group are as follows: seminoma, 37 per cent; embryonal carcinoma, 31 per cent; teratocarcinoma, 25 per cent; teratoma (adult), 2.5 per cent; choriocarcinoma, 2 per cent; and mixed tumors, 2.5 per cent. Staging is of some importance, although it may be clinically difficult to differentiate stage I and II disease. Stage I disease is confined to the testis and adnexae; stage II includes regional lymphatic involvement. Stage III refers to disseminated disease.

Seminoma has the most favorable prognosis. More than 90 per cent of the patients in most series survive five years or longer.[36, 37] Seminomas are usually in stage I or stage II at the time of diagnosis. Early spread is confined to lymphatic routes, and most of these tumors are radiosensitive. On the other hand, testicular carcinoma is usually (but not always) radioresistant, and approximately 80 per cent of these tumors are in stage II or stage III at the time of diagnosis. The five-year survival rate for embryonal carcinoma has been reported to be as low as 10 to 30 per cent[38] and as high as 75 per cent.[37]

The therapeutic approach to testicular neoplasms of germinal cell origin is outlined in Figure 3–7. Initial evaluation includes chest roentgenography with tomography, if necessary, and lymphangiography. The primary therapy for seminoma is orchiectomy and radiation therapy or radiation therapy alone;[36] for other germ cell tumors it is orchiectomy in combination with retroperitoneal lymphadenectomy or radiation therapy, or both. Guidelines for radiation therapy and extensive lymph node dissection have not been definitively established.[39]

In patients with disseminated disease, the response to cytostatic agents has been variable. Chemotherapy may be of definite benefit, and even a few "cures" in which there is no evidence of disease five or more years after treatment have been reported. At the present time, the initial therapy of choice for metastatic tumors is probably an intensive course of an alkylating agent, alternated with either methotrexate or actinomycin-D.

The following program has been used with considerable success at the University of California San Francisco Medical Center.[40] At monthly intervals the patient is treated with nitrogen mustard, 0.4

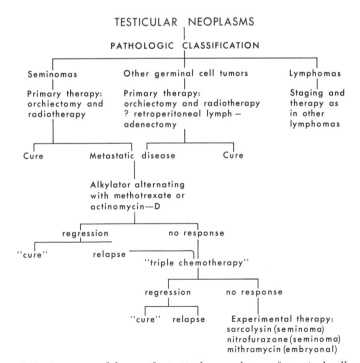

Figure 3–7   Sequence of therapy for testicular neoplasms of germinal cell origin.

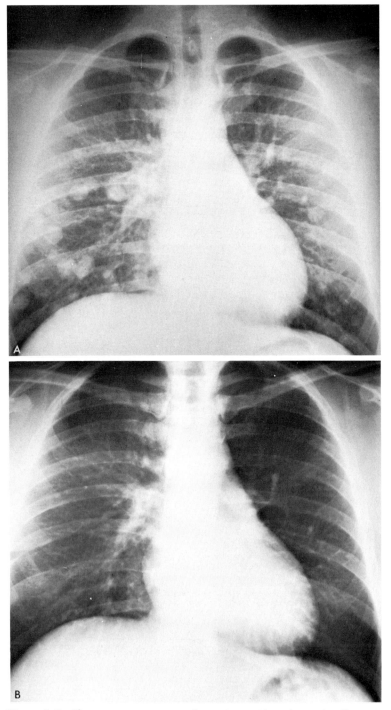

Figure 3–8 Chest roentgenograms of a patient with embryonal cell carcinoma of the testis. A: before treatment; B: after treatment with a combination of chemotherapeutic agents.

mg. per kg., alternated with either actinomycin-D, 0.5 mg. given intravenously on each of 4 successive days, or with intravenous administration of methotrexate, 25 mg. on each of 5 consecutive days. Such a program appears to be at least as good as, and probably superior to, simultaneous therapy with three agents.[39] The results of therapy in a single patient with embryonal cell carcinoma are illustrated in Figure 3–8.

In the patient whose disease fails to respond or who becomes refractory to treatment with single agents, multiple-drug therapy should be used. Many such regimens have been described in the literature; two are outlined here as examples.

1. Methotrexate, 5 mg. orally daily; chlorambucil, 10 mg. orally daily for 25 days, with actinomycin-D, 0.5 mg. intravenously daily for three 5-day courses beginning on the third, twelfth, and twenty-first days respectively.[39]

2. Methotrexate, 5 mg. orally daily; cyclophosphamide, 2 mg. per kg. orally daily; intravenous administration of vincristine, 0.025 mg. per kg. weekly.[40]

The toxic reactions associated with combination chemotherapy may be significant. They are less severe if relatively conservative drug dose levels are employed and if schedules are "individualized" by reducing or discontinuing individual drugs in the combination according to the degree of response elicited and the major form of toxicity affecting the patient. The therapeutic program is evaluated by periodic measurements of palpable masses, serial chest roentgenograms if the patient has pulmonary metastases, intravenous pyelograms in patients with retroperitoneal involvement, and all appropriate laboratory studies for hematopoietic, renal, and hepatic toxicity as well as 24-hour urinary chorionic gonadotropin titers.

There is no apparent difference in the response rate of the different types of germinal cell carcinomas to chemotherapy.

If the patient's malignancy does not respond to one of the multiple-agent regimens, experimental agents such as sarcolysin (seminoma, ref. 41), nitrofurazone (seminoma, ref. 42), or mithramycin (ref. 43) may be considered.

RENAL CELL CARCINOMA (HYPERNEPHROMA)

The primary treatment of renal cell carcinoma is surgical. Good prognostic factors include a tumor of less than 5 cm. diameter, no invasion of the capsule, absence of venous involvement, and a histologic pattern of clear cells (typical hypernephroma, ref. 44). In patients with inoperable or metastatic disease, the prognosis is grim: 72 per cent are dead within a year.[45] In patients with metastatic bone lesions, radiation therapy is useful in the palliation of pain. In con-

trast, chemotherapy with cytotoxic agents has been of only questionable value in achieving such palliation.[46] However, in 1964
Bloom[47] reported objective benefit in 20 per cent of a small group of
patients treated with a progestational agent and testosterone. These
observations were subsequently confirmed in a large series of patients by Bloom and also by other investigators.[48, 49] The use of these
hormones clinically was suggested by studies of estrogen-dependent
renal tumors in the Syrian hamster.[50]

In view of the relative benignity of treatment with these hormonal agents, they should be tried first in patients with disseminated
hypernephroma. The sequence of treatment should be progesterone
and then testosterone, although both hormones may be used together
in rapidly advancing disease.

The optimal dosage of progestational agents has not been established, but as a first approximation the schedule of Samuels[48] can be
used: medroxyprogesterone acetate (Provera), 100 mg. per day intramuscularly or a Depo preparation (Depo-Provera), 400 mg. per week.
Therapy should be continued for at least 12 weeks. In patients
failing to respond to treatment, testosterone propionate or enanthate
can be given intramuscularly in a dosage of 600 to 800 mg. per week.

Occasional responses of hypernephroma to 6-mercaptopurine[51]
and vinblastine[52] have been reported, but these cannot be considered as generally useful agents.

CARCINOMA OF THE BLADDER

The effectiveness of 5-fluorouracil in the treatment of carcinoma
of the bladder has varied widely in different reports.[53, 54] Recently, a
carefully controlled study in which the effectiveness of 5-fluorouracil
was compared to that of a placebo was reported.[55] It was clear that 5-
fluorouracil demonstrated no advantage over the placebo. Further-
more, this study demonstrated that regression of disease occurred in
some patients treated with a placebo alone, indicating that carcinoma
of the bladder does not develop in a predictably measurable manner.
This study also demonstrates the critical need for appropriate con-
trols in evaluating anticancer drugs.

REFERENCES

1. Huggins, C., Stevens, R. E., Jr., and Hodges, C. V.: Studies on prostatic cancer. II.
    The effects of castration on advanced carcinoma of the prostate gland. Arch.
    Surg., 43:209–223, 1941.
2. Alder, A., Burger, H., Davis, J., Dulmanis, A., Hudson, B., Sarfaty, G., and Straffon,
    W.: Carcinoma of prostate: Response of plasma luteinizing hormone and testos-
    terone to oestrogen therapy. Brit. Med. J., 1:28–30, 1968.

3. Arduino, L. J., and Mellinger, G. T.: Clinical trial of busulfan (NSC–750) in advanced carcinoma of prostate. Cancer Chemother. Rep., 51:295–303, 1967.
4. Carcinoma of the prostate: A continuing cooperative study. The Veterans Administration Cooperative Urological Research Group. J. Urol., 91:590–594, 1964.
5. Barber, H. R. K., and Brunschweig, A.: Treatment and results of recurrent cancer of corpus uteri in patients receiving anterior and total pelvic exenteration 1947–1963. Cancer, 22:949, 1968.
6. Truskett, I. D., and Constable, W. C.: Management of carcinoma of the corpus uteri. Amer. J. Obstet. Gynec., 101:689–694, 1968.
7. Kelly, R. M., and Baker, W. H.: Progestational agents in the treatment of carcinoma of the endometrium. New Eng. J. Med., 264:216-222, 1961.
8. Kelly, R. M., and Baker, W. H.: The role of progesterone in human endometrial cancer. Cancer Res., 25:1190–1192, 1965.
9. Kistner, R. W., Griffiths, C. T., and Craig, J. M.: Use of progestational agents in the management of endometrial cancer. Cancer, 18:1563–1579, 1965.
10. Malkasian, G. D., Jr., Mussey, E., Decker, D. G., and Johnson, C. E.: Chemotherapy of gynecologic sarcomas. Cancer Chemother. Rep., 51:507–516, 1967.
11. Maus, J. H., Mackay, E. N., and Sellers, A. H.: Cancer of the ovary. A twenty-one year study of 1,722 patients treated in the Ontario cancer clinics, 1938–1958 inclusive. Amer. J. Roent., 102:603–607, 1968.
12. Frick, H. C., Atchoo, N., Adamson, K., Jr., and Taylor, H. C., Jr.: The efficacy of chemotherapeutic agents in the management of disseminated gynecologic cancer. Review of 206 cases. Amer. J. Obstet. Gynec., 93:1112–1121, 1965.
13. Calabresi, P., and Welch, A. D.: Cytotoxic drugs, hormones, and radioactive isotopes. In Goodman, L. S., and Gilman, A. (Editors): The Pharmacological Basis of Therapeutics. Ed. 3. New York, The Macmillan Company, 1965, p. 1345.
14. Hreshchyshyn, M. M., and Holland, J. F.: Chemotherapy in patients with gynecologic cancer. Amer. J. Obstet. Gynec., 83:468–489, 1962.
15. Masterson, J. G., Calame, R. J., and Nelson, J.: A clinical study on the use of chlorambucil in the treatment of cancer of the ovary. Amer. J. Obstet. Gynec., 79:1002–1007, 1960.
16. Rundles, R. W., Laszlo, J., Garrison, F. E., Jr., and Hobson, J. B.: The antitumor spectrum of cyclophosphamide. Cancer Chemother. Rep., 16:407, 1962.
17. Frick, H. C., II, Tretter, P., Tretter, W., and Hyman, G. A.: Disseminated carcinoma of the ovary treated by L-phenylalanine mustard. Cancer, 21:508–513, 1968.
18. Greenspan, E. M., and Fieber, M.: Combination chemotherapy of advanced ovarian carcinoma with the antimetabolite, methotrexate, and the alkylating agent, Thiotepa. J. Mount Sinai Hospital, 29:48–62, 1962.
19. Hreshchyshyn, M. M.: A critical review of chemotherapy in the treatment of ovarian carcinoma. Clin. Obst. Gynec., 4:885–900, 1961.
20. Mathé, G., Dausset, J., Hervet, E., Amiel, J. L., Colombani, J., and Brule, G.: Immunological studies in patients with placental choriocarcinoma. J. Nat. Cancer Inst., 33:193–208, 1964.
21. Hertz, R., Lewis, J., Jr., and Lipsett, M. B.: Five years' experience with the chemotherapy of metastatic choriocarcinoma and related trophoblastic tumors in women. Amer. J. Obstet. Gynec., 82:631–640, 1961.
22. Hertig, A. T., and Gore, H. M.: Tumors of the female sex organs. In Atlas of Tumor Pathology. Washington, D.C., Armed Forces Institute of Pathology, 1956, Section IX, Fasc. 33, pp. 7–15.
23. Delfs, E.: Chorionic gonadotrophin determinations in patients with hydatidiform mole and choriocarcinoma. Ann. New York Acad. Sci., 80:125–139, 1959.
24. Hertz, R., Ross, G. T., and Lipsett, M. B.: Primary chemotherapy of nonmetastatic trophoblastic disease in women. Amer. J. Obstet. Gynec., 86:808–814, 1963.
25. Bagshawe, K. D.: Trophoblastic tumors: Chemotherapy and developments. Brit. Med. J., 2:1303–1307, 1963.
26. Li, M. C., Hertz, R., and Spencer, D. B.: Effect of methotrexate therapy upon choriocarcinoma and chorioadenoma. Proc. Soc. Exp. Biol. Med., 93:361–366, 1956.
27. Johnson, F. D., Jacobs, E. M., and Silliphant, W. M.: Trophoblastic tumors of the uterus. Problems of methotrexate therapy. California Med., 108:1–13, 1968.

28. Wide, L.: An immunological method for the assay of human chorionic gonadotropin. Acta Endocrinol., 41(Suppl.):70, 1962.
29. Li, M. C., Hertz, R., and Bergenstal, D. M.: Therapy of choriocarcinoma and related trophoblastic tumors with folic acid and purine antagonists. New Eng. J. Med., 259:66–74, 1958.
30. Ross, G. T., Goldstein, D. P., Hertz, R., Lipsett, M. B., and Odell, W. D.: Sequential use of methotrexate and actinomycin-D in the treatment of metastatic choriocarcinoma and related trophoblastic diseases in women. Amer. J. Obstet. Gynec., 93:223–229, 1965.
31. Li, M. C.: Management of choriocarcinoma and related tumors of uterus and testis. Med. Clin. N. Amer., 45:661–676, 1961.
32. Hertz, R., Lipsett, M. B., and Moy, R. H.: Effect of vincaleukoblastine on metastatic choriocarcinoma and related trophoblastic tumors in women. Cancer Res., 20:1050–1053, 1960.
33. Abell, M. R., and Holtz, F.: Testicular and paratesticular neoplasms in patients 60 years of age and older. Cancer, 21:852–870, 1968.
34. Dixon, F. J., and Moore, R. A.: Testicular tumors. A clinicopathological study. Cancer, 6:427–454, 1953.
35. Patton, J. F., Hewitt, C. B., and Mallis, N.: Diagnosis and treatment of tumors of the testis. J.A.M.A., 171:2194–2198, 1959.
36. Maier, J. G., Sulak, M. H., and Mittemeyer, B. T.: Seminoma of the testis: Analysis of treatment success and failure. Amer. J. Roent., 102:596–602, 1968.
37. Patton, J. F., Seitzman, D. N., and Zone, R. A.: Diagnosis and treatment of testicular tumors. Amer. J. Surg., 99:525–602, 1960.
38. Friedman, M., and Di Rienzo, A. J.: Treatment of trophocarcinoma (embryonal carcinoma) of the testis. Radiology, 80:550–565, 1963.
39. Whitmore, W. F., Jr.: Some experiences with retroperitoneal lymph node dissection and chemotherapy in management of testis neoplasms. Brit. J. Urol., 34:436–447, 1962.
40. Jacobs, E. M., Johnson, F. D., and Wood, D. A.: Stage III metastatic malignant testicular tumors. Cancer, 19:1697–1704, 1966.
41. Blokhin, N., Larionov, L., Perevodchikova, N., Chebotareva, L., and Mekulova, N.: Clinical experiences with sarcolysin in neoplastic diseases. Ann. New York Acad. Sci., 68:1128, 1958.
42. Marshall, M., Jr., Johnson, S. H., III, and Price, S. E., Jr.: Metastatic seminoma of testis treated by oral nitrofurazone (Furacin) and radiotherapy. J. Urol., 91:392–395, 1964.
43. Brown, J. H., and Kennedy, B. J.: Mithramycin in the treatment of disseminated testicular neoplasms. New Eng. J. Med., 272:111–118, 1965.
44. Kay, S.: Renal carcinoma. A 10-year study. Amer. J. Clin. Path., 50:428–432, 1968.
45. Royce, R. K., and Tormey, A. R.: Malignant tumors of the renal parenchyma in adults. J. Urol., 74:23–35, 1955.
46. Woodruff, M. W., Wagle, D., Gailani, S. D., and Jones, R., Jr.: The current status of chemotherapy for advanced renal carcinoma. J. Urol., 97:611–618, 1967.
47. Bloom, H. J. G.: Hormone treatment of renal tumors. Experimental and clinical observations. In Riches, E. (Editor): Tumors of the Kidney and Ureter. Baltimore, The Williams & Wilkins Co., 1964, p. 311.
48. Samuels, M. L., Sullivan, P., and Howe, C. D.: Medroxyprogesterone acetate in the treatment of renal cell carcinoma (hypernephroma). Cancer, 22:525–532, 1968.
49. Talley, R. W., Moorhead, E. L., II, Tucker, W. G., San Diego, E. L., and Brennan, M. J.: Treatment of metastatic hypernephroma. J.A.M.A., 207:322–328, 1969.
50. Kirkham, H.: Estrogen-induced tumors of the kidney. III. Growth characteristics in the Syrian hamster. National Cancer Institute Monograph No. 1. Washington, D.C., United States Department of Health, Education and Welfare, 1959, p. 1.
51. Lemon, H. M., Miller, D. M., Smith, J., and Walker, E. E.: Remission of metastases of erythropoietin-secreting renal cell adenocarcinoma after 6-mercaptopurine (NSC–755) therapy. Cancer Chemother. Rep., 36:49–54, 1964.
52. Smart, C. R., Rochlin, D. B., Nahum, A. M., Silva, A., and Wagner, D.: Clinical experience with vinblastine sulfate (NSC–49842) in squamous cell carcinoma and other malignancies. Cancer Chemother. Rep., 34:31–45, 1964.

53. Deren, T. L., and Wilson, W. L.: Use of 5-fluorouracil in treatment of bladder carcinomas. J. Urol., 83:390–393, 1960.
54. Glenn, J. F., Hunt, L. D., and Lathem, J. E.: Chemotherapy of bladder carcinoma with 5-fluorouracil. Cancer Chemother. Rep., 27:67–69, 1963.
55. Prout, G. R., Bross, I. J. D., Slack, N. H., and Ausman, R. K.: Carcinoma of the bladder, 5-fluorouracil and the critical role of a placebo. A cooperative Group Report. I. Cancer, 22:926–931, 1968.

Additional Recent Bibliography Not Cited in Text

56. Rubin, P.: Cancer of the urogenital tract: Prostatic cancer. Introduction. J.A.M.A., 209:1695–1705, 1969.
57. Wider, J. A., Marshall, J. R., Bardin, C. W., Lipsett, M. B., and Ross, G. T.: Sustained remissions after chemotherapy for primary ovarian cancers containing choriocarcinoma. New Eng. J. Med., 280:1439, 1969.
58. Boctor, Z. N., Kurohara, S. S., Badib, A. O., and Murphy, G. P.: Current results from therapy of testicular tumors. Cancer, 24:870–875, 1969.
59. Ansfield, F. J., Korbitz, B. C., Davis, H. L., and Ramirez, G.: Triple drug therapy in testicular tumors. Cancer, 24:442–446, 1969.
60. Jacobs, E. M.: Combination chemotherapy of metastatic testicular germinal cell tumors and soft part sarcomas. Cancer, 25:324–332, 1970.
61. Samuels, M. L., and Howe, C. D.: Vinblastine in the management of testicular cancer. Cancer, 25:1009–1017, 1970.
62. Monto, R. W., Talley, R. W., Caldwell, M. J., Levin, W. C., and Guest, M. M.: Observations on the mechanism of hemorrhagic toxicity in mithramycin (NSC 24559) therapy. Cancer Res., 29:697–704, 1969.
63. Rafla, S.: Renal cell carcinoma. Natural history and results of treatment. Cancer, 25:26–40, 1970.

CHAPTER 4

CARCINOMA OF THE BREAST

CARCINOMA OF THE FEMALE BREAST

INCIDENCE

In no area of cancer therapy is there more confusion or difference of opinion about the modalities and sequence of treatment than in carcinoma of the breast. Despite long experience, intensive study, and a voluminous literature, no general principles of management have been universally adopted in the treatment of this neoplasm. This tumor is the commonest malignancy and the leading cause of death in American women in the middle of life.

The annual incidence of carcinoma of the breast in the United States is approximately 70 per 100,000 women, and the mortality rate is 24 per 100,000.[1, 2a] There are now 65,000 new cases and 28,000 deaths annually. Unfortunately the annual incidence of breast cancer seems to be increasing in this country just as it is in Scandinavia, Wales, and England. The factors involved in this increase are not known. However, this increase is not simply a reflection of the increased longevity of the female population. One consequence of this increased incidence is that the annual mortality from breast cancer (deaths per 100,000 female population) has not changed in recent years despite the improvements in medical management. Misinterpretation of this finding has resulted in the gloomy conclusion that there has been little progress in the therapy of breast cancer in the past three decades.[2a] In fact, the chances of cure for the individual patient with breast cancer today are considerably better than they were in the past—earlier detection is the probable explanation.

Factors that are thought to have some bearing on the development of breast cancer include previous ovariectomy, nulliparity, and a family history of breast cancer.[2b–4]

The management of sarcomas and related mesenchymal tumors of the female breast represents a problem distinct from that of the more common mammary carcinoma. The reader may wish to consult pertinent reviews.[5, 6]

PREDICTION OF RESPONSE TO THERAPY

It is difficult to define precisely all the factors that are useful in predicting response to therapy, but some have been clearly identified. These are as follows:

1. Extent of spread of malignancy at the time of diagnosis
2. Length of time that has elapsed between mastectomy and the first detectable recurrence
3. Site of metastasis
4. Age of the patient

Foremost among the predictive factors is the extent of spread at the time of surgery. At the present time, the reported 5-year survival rate for patients with early (stage I) carcinoma (axillary nodes not involved) at the time of "standard" radical mastectomy is almost 90 per cent; the reported survival rates range from less than 50 per cent to about 60 per cent for patients with involved axillary nodes.

Another prognostic factor is the rate of growth of the tumor as gauged by the free interval, the period between radical mastectomy and the time of diagnosis of metastasis. If this interval exceeds one year, the patient has a better than average chance of responding to therapy for metastatic breast cancer.[7] In such patients, the duration of response is often long. The "free interval" is another way of expressing the ancient clinical observation that slowly growing malignant tumors kill more slowly than rapidly growing tumors.

A third prognostic consideration is the site of metastasis. Metastatic disease in the soft tissues including the breast, regional lymph nodes, pleural cavity, skin, or bone, carries a better prognosis than metastasis to the abdominal and thoracic viscera or to the brain. This phenomenon merely reflects the fact that a tumor involving a vital organ is more apt to be lethal than a tumor involving a site not essential for life.

It is now well established that hormonal treatment of breast cancer is more effective in elderly than in young women. For example, the response to estrogens tends to be better in postmenopausal patients of advanced age than in recently menopausal ones. In advanced disease, previous response to castration or other hormonal manipulation may also be useful in predicting the response to other ablative hormonal therapy.

Despite occasional reports to the contrary, it is unlikely that the histologic features of carcinoma of the breast have any significant prognostic import. Similarly, the host of biochemical analyses that have been used in an attempt to predict the response to endocrine manipulation have been disappointing. (See the review by Crowley, ref. 8.) It is sufficient to note that none of them has achieved a place in the routine management of the patient with breast cancer.

THERAPY OF RECURRENT OR METASTATIC DISEASE

In the treatment of carcinoma of the breast, it is important to distinguish between definitive therapy of the primary lesion and treatment of recurrent or disseminated disease. The management of carcinoma localized to a single breast and its lymphatic drainage falls within the province of the surgeon and the radiation therapist. It is not within the realm of the chemotherapist. Considerable controversy exists as to the extent of surgery and the use of radiation therapy. The reader may wish to consult the excellent recent reviews of the successes and failures of current initial therapy of carcinoma of the breast.[9-13a, 13b] The discussion in the present chapter is concerned with management of recurrent or metastatic disease.

Evaluation of the Response to Therapy

What criteria does the physician apply when evaluating the effectiveness of therapy? Obviously, objective parameters of tumor response are best. Weight gain, an increase in hematocrit, and a sense of well-being are important guides to therapy, but the evaluation must be based on the measurable response of the tumor.

The following three parameters of response are used:
1. Measurable tumors become smaller.
2. Osteolytic lesions recalcify.
3. No new lesions appear during the period of treatment.

The Cooperative Breast Cancer Group (a group supported by the National Institutes of Health) has stipulated that two physicians not involved directly in the care of the patient must agree on these parameters of response before declaring that an experimental drug has a beneficial effect. This requirement is obviously not practical in the management of most patients, but the principle is sound. A placebo effect of a drug is undesirable in a disease so responsive to therapy.

Program of Sequential Hormonal Manipulation and Chemotherapy

Figure 4–1 indicates one program of sequential therapy for recurrent carcinoma of the breast. A number of other, alternative

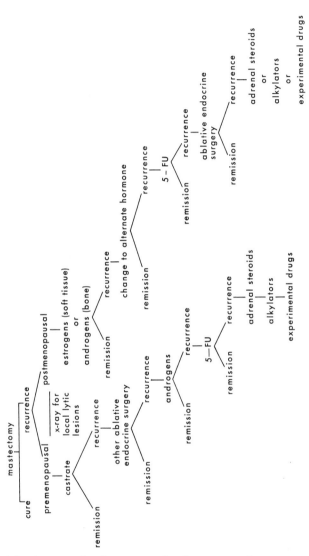

Figure 4-1 An example of a program for the sequential management of metastatic carcinoma of the breast.

therapeutic programs that reflect the opinions of other investigators are available. The most useful agents are listed in Table 4–1. An alternative sequence recommended by one authority consists of castration if the patient is premenopausal and, first, a trial of hormonal therapy, then secondary hormonal therapy, and finally chemotherapy —rarely followed by endocrine ablative procedures for those few patients who have previously responded to castration and whose disease is progressing and no longer responding to drug therapy.[13a]

Before embarking on a discussion of the chemotherapeutic program, it is worthwhile stressing certain general principles in treating the patient with disseminated carcinoma of the breast.

First, *only one course of therapy at a time* is employed. The exception to this rule is the irradiation of lytic lesions of weight-bearing bone in combination with other treatment.

Second, *therapy is changed only if disease is advancing*, not, as a rule, if it is static.

Third, after a given therapeutic program has been discontinued, the patient should be observed for a while to ascertain the effects of withdrawing the drug ("*remission of withdrawal*") before a new program is started. The "remission of withdrawal" or "rebound regression" is most likely to occur in patients who have had a beneficial effect from estrogen therapy. The response rate in those patients who have failed to respond to estrogens or who have been treated with androgens is only about 2 or 3 per cent.

Finally, *contraceptive pills are contraindicated* in the young

TABLE 4–1   *Agents Useful in the Treatment of Carcinoma of the Breast*

Class of Compounds	Drug	Route of Administration	Usual Dosage
Androgens	Testosterone enanthate (Delatestryl)	I.M.	200–300 mg./week
	Fluoxymesterone (Halotestin)	Oral	10–30 mg./day
Estrogens	Diethylstilbestrol	Oral	5–15 mg./day
Antimetabolites	5-Fluorouracil	I.V.	10–15 mg./kg. once weekly
Alkylating agents	Nitrogen mustard	I.V.	0.2–0.5 mg./kg. in a single course
	Chlorambucil (Leukeran)	Oral	2–6 mg./day
	Cyclophosphamide (Cytoxan)	Oral	50–150 mg./day
		I.V.	20–40 mg./kg. in a single course
Adrenal steroids	Prednisone	Oral	20–100 mg./day
	Prednisolone	I.V.	20–100 mg./day

patient because they introduce another hormonal variable and, in some instances, may cause exacerbation of disease.

The Premenopausal Patient

Selection of the mode of hormonal manipulation in managing recurrent breast carcinoma depends on the patient's menopausal status. Patients who have menses or are within one year of the menopause are considered to be premenopausal.

OVARIECTOMY. The first approach in the premenopausal patient with metastatic breast cancer is castration. Ovariectomy is performed to remove ovarian hormones that have a stimulatory effect on the growth of breast cancer: androgen, progestin, and estrogen. Between 30 and 40 per cent of premenopausal patients are benefited by ovariectomy. The mean duration of response approximates 15 months. If the patient is an acceptable operative risk, surgical castration is preferable to ovarian irradiation. If the patient is not a surgical candidate, an x-ray dose in the range of 1200 to 1800 rads will effectively destroy ovarian function, although at a slower rate than ovariectomy.[14]

Castration by either method should be reserved for premenopausal patients with evidence of advancing disease for several reasons. There is no convincing evidence that "prophylatic" castration at the time of intial surgery prolongs survival.[8, 15, 16] Such prophylactic castration will obviously involve a small number of patients already cured by primary surgery. Finally, the response to castration is useful in predicting the response to subsequent hormonal therapy, and this guide is lost by prophylactic ovariectomy.

In the castrated patient who suffers a relapse and has unequivocal evidence of progressive disease, three major therapeutic alternatives are open to the physician: further ablative surgery (adrenalectomy or hypophysectomy), androgen therapy, or chemotherapy. The choice among these alternatives must be determined by the circumstances of the individual case. In Figure 4–1 further ablative surgery is designated as the first choice because of the high response rate. However, in patients failing to respond to castration, subsequent ablative surgery has a relatively small chance of success and alternatives should be considered.

ADRENALECTOMY AND HYPOPHYSECTOMY. Adrenalectomy or hypophysectomy can be expected to benefit approximately 30 per cent of those patients who respond to castration, but only 10 per cent of those who do not respond; therefore, as pointed out earlier, the response to castration is a useful guide to subsequent therapy. In a compilation of published reports totaling over 2,000 cases of adrenalectomy for advanced carcinoma of the breast, objective remissions exceeding 4 to 6 months occurred in approximately one-third of the

patients so treated.[8] Hypophysectomy is not superior to adrenalectomy either in rate or in duration of remissions.[9] Whether hypophysectomy or adrenalectomy should be performed depends on the
experience of the surgeons at any given institution. There is no doubt
that an adrenalectomized patient is considerably easier to manage
than one who has undergone hypophysectomy; consequently, in
most institutions adrenalectomy has replaced hypophysectomy.

An additional consideration in regard to hypophysectomy is the
observation that in unselected patients with advanced breast cancer,
replacement therapy alone (cortisol, 30 mg. daily, and triiodothyro-
nine, 50 mg. daily) produced a higher rate of tumor regression than
did hypophysectomy and replacement therapy.[13a]

After adrenalectomy, replacement therapy is required. Cortisol,
25 to 50 mg. per day by mouth, and fluorohydrocortisone, 0.1 mg.
every other day, usually suffice. During periods of stress the dose
should be increased. In most large treatment centers the operative
mortality rate for adrenalectomy is 5 per cent or less. However, in
terminally ill patients the mortality rate is much higher, and alternative methods of therapy should be used. Symptomatic cerebral metastatic disease and incapacitating respiratory insufficiency are the
other major contraindications to adrenalectomy.

A question often asked is whether there is any place in the
treatment of advanced breast cancer for simultaneous castration and
adrenalectomy as opposed to sequential therapy. The answer, simply
stated, is "no."[8, 17, 18] How adrenalectomy works is a question unan-
swered since the original observations of Huggins and Bergenstal[19]
on the effectiveness of adrenalectomy in advanced breast cancer.
The rationale often given is that bilateral adrenalectomy removes a
significant source of the production of estrogens and perhaps progestins. It has been suggested, however, that its effectiveness may also
result at least in part from the replacement therapy with adrenal
hormones. At the moment, one must admit that the mechanisms by
which endocrine manipulations affect hormone-responsive breast
cancers remain obscure.

ANDROGENS.   The premenopausal castrated patient who fails to
respond to adrenalectomy or hypophysectomy, or who relapses after
initially responding, should be considered for androgen therapy.
There are some patients, however, to whom the virilizing effects of
androgens are intolerable, and alternative therapy such as chemotherapy is preferable. Beneficial responses to androgens may be anticipated in roughly 15 to 20 per cent of the patients.[20] The median
duration of the response approximates 9 months. Testosterone pro-
prionate, 50 to 100 mg. intramuscularly three times weekly, testosterone enanthate, 200 to 300 mg. weekly, or fluoxymesterone by
mouth, 10 to 20 mg. per day, usually suffices.

A number of other compounds resembling testosterone have

been recommended at one time or another as being superior. These include Δ^1-testololactone, 2α-methyldihydrotestosterone, and 17α-methyl-19-nortestosterone. In general, they have not lived up to their initial promise, because of low antitumor activity, hepatotoxicity, fluid-retaining activity, or other disadvantages.

The mechanism of action of androgens in breast cancer is uncertain. They affect secretion by certain endocrine organs including the ovaries, adrenals, pituitary, and thyroid. They are generally thought to be antiestrogenic. Recent studies have indicated that androgens can accumulate in certain animal and human breast tumors.[21]

The most common undesirable primary effect of androgens is virilization. The acquired facial hirsutism is rarely reversible. Common side effects include fluid retention and erythrocytosis. The most serious complication is hypercalcemia, which occurs in 7 to 10 per cent of treated women. This complication demands immediate cessation of androgen administration and the institution of a high fluid intake and adrenal corticosteroids.

A number of experimental protocols for advanced breast cancer that utilize antimetabolites alone or in combination with androgens have been described recently.[22, 23] More exciting yet is the advent of new agents that are said to have pronounced antitumor activity and little in the way of virilizing side effects; for example, $7\beta,17\alpha$-dimethyltestosterone.[13a] These agents are still experimental and are not generally available, but hold high promise for the future.

5-FLUOROURACIL. Subsequent relapses after androgen therapy may be treated sequentially with chemotherapy. As our experience with 5-FU has increased, the drug-associated morbidity and mortality have been reduced; the latter is now well under 2 per cent. The program at the University of California, San Francisco, is to give a single weekly injection, 15 mg. per kg., or rarely 20 mg. per kg., until either there is an objective response or gastrointestinal or hematologic toxicity requires a reduction in the dose or cessation of administration of the drug.[24] Nine of 13 adequately treated patients showed an objective response of greater than 50 per cent.[24] Other more vigorous treatment schedules have been described by investigators at the University of Wisconsin.[25] The reported response rates with the standard regimen of 5-FU have varied between 16 and 30 per cent. This wide range reflects the variability in patient populations, the stage of the disease, and the criteria of response used in different studies.

ADRENOCORTICOSTEROIDS. Once the preceding maneuvers of endocrine manipulation and 5-FU therapy have been exhausted, there are still several therapeutic possibilities. A small number of patients may be expected to respond briefly to adrenocorticosteroids or to alkylating agents. The rationale for the use of adrenocorticosteroids is the suppression of sex hormone production by the adrenal glands and inhibition of the pituitary. Whether this is, in fact, the basis of the beneficial effect is not known. Adequate therapy means the equivalent of at least 20 mg. of prednisone per day. The appropriate measures to avoid hypokalemia and gastric ulceration are included as part of standard therapy.

The response rate of adrenocorticosteroids after castration approximates 25 per cent, and the median duration of remission is roughly 5 months.[8, 9] Symptomatic improvement occurs more often than objective tumor regression. Because objective improvement is generally of short duration and because of the troublesome side effects of these steroids, their use should generally be restricted to the patient who has failed to respond to other endocrine manipulations and to chemotherapy. Corticosteroids are also useful in the treatment of hypercalcemia occurring either spontaneously or in association with androgen or estrogen therapy[26] and in the treatment of patients with symptomatic cerebral metastases.

ALKYLATING AGENTS.   Alkylating agents occasionally produce objective responses in patients with disseminated carcinoma of the breast. Chlorambucil can be used, 2 to 6 mg. per day by mouth, or nitrogen mustard, 0.2 to 0.5 mg. per kg. given intravenously in a single course.

Intrapleural administration of nitrogen mustard (0.2 to 0.4 mg. per kg.) or Thiotepa (10 to 50 mg.) and intra-abdominal administration of Thiotepa given every 14 to 21 days are often successful in managing intractable malignant effusions (see Chap. 14). It should be stressed that a few isolated lesions of bone or skin often respond well to local x-irradiation and are not necessarily indications for systemic therapy.

ILLUSTRATIVE CASE HISTORY: CARCINOMA OF THE BREAST

The clinical course and response to therapy of a premenopausal woman are outlined in Figure 4-2.

The patient was in good health until, at the age of 32 (November 1959), a radical mastectomy was performed for carcinoma of the left breast. Eight of 20 lymph nodes were found to be involved by the malignancy, and postoperative x-irradiation was given to the left axillary area. The patient remained free of symptoms until June 1966 (about 6½ years), when a mass was found in the right breast. She was still having menses at this time. No other evidence of malignant disease was found. A right radical mastectomy was performed.

In *March 1967*, the patient complained of increasing shortness of breath with exertion. A chest roentgenogram revealed bilateral pleural effusions. Malignant cells were found in aspirated fluid. Other radiologic and labora-

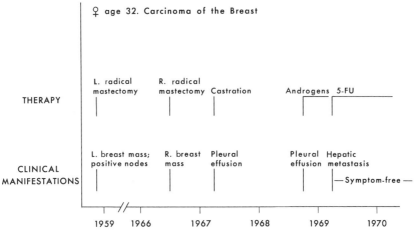

Figure 4-2 Summary of the clinical course and response to therapy of a premenopausal patient. See case history.

tory studies were within normal limits, except for the slightly elevated serum alkaline phosphatase level.

In *April 1967*, a bilateral oophorectomy was performed and the patient made an uneventful postoperative recovery. Within 5 weeks after surgery, the small amount of residual pleural fluid had disappeared and the serum alkaline phosphatase had returned to a normal level. For 17 months (May 1967 to September 1968) the patient felt entirely well and her performance status was normal. In *September 1968*, pleural effusions recurred; again the pleural fluid contained malignant cells. No other abnormalities were found.

Therapy with fluoxymesterone, 20 mg. daily by mouth, was begun. By late *November 1968*, the pleural fluid had disappeared. The patient noted slight oiliness of the skin and a few comedones with this androgen therapy, but no alopecia, facial hair growth, or change in libido. The patient continued to take oral androgens with good effect for almost 6 months, until *February 1969*, when she noted weight loss and complained of anorexia. Shortly thereafter, increasing anemia and jaundice developed and her clinical condition began to deteriorate rapidly. Liver metastasis was documented by a radioisotopic scan and percutaneous needle biopsy.

The patient was judged too ill to be a candidate for adrenalectomy, and treatment with 5-FU was begun in late February. Because of serious impairment of hepatic function, the 5-FU dose was smaller than usual—500 to 700 mg. given intravenously once weekly. Within 3 weeks a dramatic improvement was apparent: the jaundice disappeared, and abnormal elevations of hepatic enzymes returned to normal. The patient's appetite improved and she began to gain weight. Within 6 weeks after initiating 5-FU therapy her anemia improved without transfusion.

The patient continued to receive weekly injections of 5-FU, 500 to 1000 mg., until February 1970. Except for transient mild stomatitis associated with the 5-FU therapy, she has been asymptomatic and functioning normally.

COMMENT: This young woman underwent a radical mastectomy for carcinoma of the left breast. About 6½ years later a tumor was diagnosed in the right breast. In was not certain whether the second lesion represented metastatic disease after a long "free interval" or whether it was a second primary tumor. A right radical mastectomy was performed. However, 9 months later metastatic disease was found in the pleural cavity. The patient's subsequent course over a period of 3 years was characterized by metastatic disease of the pleural cavity and liver, and sequential excellent responses to castration, androgens, and 5-FU therapy.

The Postmenopausal Patient

ESTROGENS. The sequence of therapy for patients more than 5 years postmenopausal is outlined in Figure 4–1. Estrogens are the initial therapy of choice, and a response rate of approximately 20 to 30 per cent can be anticipated, with a median duration of response of approximately 12 to 15 months. The response rate is somewhat better in patients with involvement of soft tissues and pulmonary or pleural metastases than in those with bone and visceral metastases. The response rate is higher in elderly women and is somewhat lower in women recently menopausal.

The use of estrogens in cancer of the breast[27] followed the observations of Huggins[28] that diethylstilbestrol was useful in the treatment of cancer of the prostate. The mechanism of action of estrogens in postmenopausal cancer of the breast is still unknown, despite intensive study. It is paradoxical that estrogens, which stimulate acinar and ductal development of the mammary gland and which may cause exacerbation of breast cancer in the premenopausal patient, are so frequently effective in its management in the postmenopausal patient. Elwood Jensen[29] and his collaborators have recently identified a receptor for estradiol in breast tissue cells.[29] Such studies at the subcellular level may eventually elucidate the effects of estrogenic hormones.

Diethylstilbestrol was among the first synthetic estrogens introduced and remains the standard preparation. Therapy should be initiated at the level of 15 mg. per day. The dose can subsequently be reduced when the desired effect is achieved and if side effects are poorly tolerated. Side effects include nausea, fluid retention, breast engorgement, and vaginal bleeding. In approximately 3 per cent of the treated patients, hypercalcemia is a complication, requiring abrupt cessation of therapy.[30]

ANDROGENS. In those patients who fail to respond to estrogens or who respond and then relapse, androgen therapy is the next step. A response rate of 10 to 15 per cent may be anticipated, with a median duration of response approaching 9 months. The longer the period elapsed since the menopause, the better the chances of a good response to androgens. There is suggestive evidence that androgens may be preferable to estrogens as initial therapy in patients with bone metastases. Both types of hormones may produce hypercalcemia,[30, 31] although it is likely that androgens must first be metabolized to estrogenic compounds before they result in abnormalities of calcium metabolism.[32] If hypercalcemia occurs, the hormone should be withdrawn and adrenocorticosteroid therapy begun.

5-FLUOROURACIL AND OTHER PROCEDURES. After estrogen and androgen treatment is exhausted, the therapeutic sequence is that outlined in Figure 4–1: 5-FU, further ablative surgery, adrenocorticosteroids, alkylating agents, or experimental drugs. The sequence in which 5-FU and ablative surgery should be used is not yet definitely established. Nonandrogenic progestational compounds have been used in advanced breast cancer in limited trials.[33, 34] Although occasional good responses have been observed in postmenopausal patients, the results have generally been disappointing. Progestational agents cannot be recommended for routine therapy.

ILLUSTRATIVE CASE HISTORY: CARCINOMA OF THE BREAST

The clinical course and response to therapy of a postmenopausal woman are outlined in Figure 4–3.

In *August 1967*, the patient noted a mass in the upper outer quadrant of her right breast. This lesion was examined by her physician but biopsy was not performed until *March 1968*, when a diagnosis of carcinoma was made. A right radical mastectomy was performed, and all axillary lymph nodes exam-

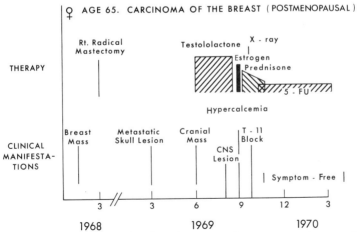

Figure 4–3 Summary of the clinical course and response to therapy of a postmenopausal patient. See case history.

ined were said to be negative for carcinoma. No postoperative irradiation was given.

In *March 1969*, one year after surgery, the patient noted a lump in the left occipitoparietal area, and skull x-ray films were interpreted as showing evidence of metastatic disease.

In *June 1969*, when the patient was first seen at the University of California Hospitals, San Francisco, she was 65 years of age, obese, and in her sixteenth year after menopause. There was no evidence of local recurrence of breast carcinoma. She complained of lumbar pain, but the findings of a neurologic examination were normal, and there was no bone tenderness. A cranial mass was noted. X-ray films of the bones revealed a questionable lytic lesion of the right humerus. The serum calcium was within normal limits, but the serum alkaline phosphatase was slightly elevated. Therapy with testololactone, 250 mg. 4 times a day, was begun.

On *August 14, 1969*, the patient re-entered the hospital because of bone pain. Roentgenologic studies revealed progressive lytic lesions of the skull (Fig. 4-4) and humerus and involvement of the lower thoracic and lumbar

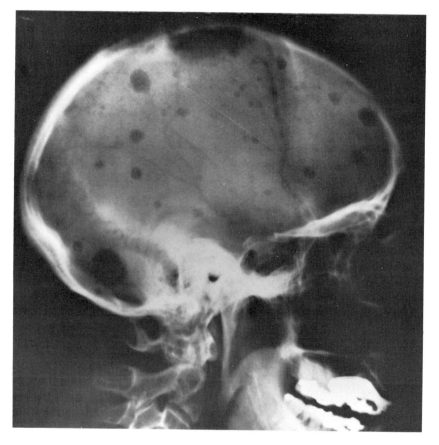

Figure 4-4 Skull roentgenogram in postmenopausal patient showing osteolytic lesions from metastatic carcinoma of the breast. See case history.

vertebrae. A radioisotopic brain scan revealed a large area of increased uptake over the left parietal area consistent with cerebral metastatic disease.

Testololactone was discontinued and therapy with stilbestrol, 5 mg. per day, was started. Within 8 days after beginning estrogen therapy, the serum calcium rose to 13.7 mg. per 100 ml. and then to 15.4 (normal, 9.2 to 10.8 mg. per 100 ml.). Estrogen therapy was immediately discontinued, and the patient was placed on a program including hydration, low calcium diet, oral sodium phosphate, and prednisone (20 mg. 4 times per day). Within 5 days, the calcium had fallen to 12.5 mg. per 100 ml. and by 7 days to 9.4 mg. per 100 ml. Prednisone was gradually reduced in amount and eventually discontinued. During this period, lumbar pain increased and a myelogram revealed a partial block of the T11 vertebra. Radiation therapy was begun, with neurosurgeons and radiation therapists working as a team.

On *October 4, 1969*, therapy was started with 5-FU, initially 7.5 mg. per kg. once weekly and subsequently 10 to 15 mg. per kg. per week. Within 5 days after the initiation of therapy the patient reported decreased bone pain; by 18 days there was radiologic evidence of bone healing. In *March 1970*, treatment was begun under an experimental protocol that included 5-FU, vincristine, and prednisone. At present the patient feels well, the bone lesions are almost completely healed, and the serum calcium is normal.

COMMENT: This postmenopausal woman with carcinoma of the breast was treated initially with an androgen for metastatic disease to bone. Disease progressed while she was under this treatment and estrogen therapy was started. Hypercalcemia developed shortly thereafter. An elevated serum calcium concentration responded to hydration, sodium phosphate, prednisone, and withdrawal of estrogens. After 5-FU therapy was started, the metastatic lesions of bone calcified.

CARCINOMA OF THE MALE BREAST

Cancer of the breast in the male is rare and relatively little experience in its management has accumulated.[35] With the exception of Klinefelter's syndrome, there is no clear-cut predisposing condition for the development of carcinoma of the male breast.[36] The most reliable form of therapy for disseminated breast cancer in males (excluding patients with Klinefelter's syndrome) appears to be castration.[37] In small series of patients, adrenalectomy has been beneficial in approximately 40 per cent[19, 38] Adrenocorticosteroids and progestins may occasionally be useful.[39]

REFERENCES

1. End Results in Cancer: Report No. 2. United States Department of Health, Education and Welfare, Public Health Service. Washington, D.C., Government Printing Office Publication No. 1149, 1964.

2a. Shimkin, M. B.: End results in cancer of the breast. Cancer, 20:1039, 1967.

2b. Bailar, J. C., King, H., and Mason, M. J.: Cancer Rates and Risks. United States Department of Health, Education and Welfare, Public Health Service. Washington, D.C., Government Printing Office Publication No. 1148, 1964.

3. Logan, W. P. D.: Marriage and childbearing in relation to cancer of the breast and uterus. Lancet, 2:1199–1202, 1953.

4. Woolf, C. M.: Investigations on Genetic Aspects of Carcinoma of the Stomach and Breast. Berkeley, University of California Press, 1955, p. 265.

5. Norris, H. J., and Taylor, H. B.: Sarcomas and related mesenchymal tumors of the breast. Cancer, 22:22–28, 1968.

6. Jernstrom, P., and Sether, J. M.: Primary lymphosarcoma of the mammary gland. J.A.M.A., 201:503–506, 1967.

7. Fairgriev, J.: Selective criteria for surgical removal of the endocrine glands in advanced breast cancer. Surg. Gynec. Obst., 120:371–385, 1965.

8. Crowley, L. G.: Current status of the management of patients with endocrine-sensitive tumors. Part 1. Introduction and carcinoma of the breast. California Med., 110:43, 1969.

9. Moore, F. D., Woodrow, S. I., Aliapoulious, M. A., and Wilson, R. E.: Carcinoma of the breast. A decade of new results with old concepts. New Eng. J. Med., 277:293, 1967.

10. Breast Cancer. Combined clinical staff conference at the National Institutes of Health. Ann. Intern. Med., 63:321–341, 1965.

11. Lewison, E. F., Montague, A. C. W., and Kuller, L.: Breast cancer treated at the Johns Hopkins Hospital, 1951–1956. Cancer, 19:1359–1368, 1966.

12. Fletcher, G. H., Montague, E. D., and White, E. C.: Evaluation of irradiation of the peripheral lymphatics in conjunction with radical mastectomy for cancer of the breast. Cancer, 21:791–797, 1968.

13a. Gordan, G. A.: Progress in the treatment of advanced breast cancer. California Med., 111:38, 1969.

13b. Haimov, M., Kark, A. E., and Lesnick, G. J.: Carcinoma of the breast. Thirty years' experience with radical mastectomy. Amer. J. Surg., 115:341–348, 1968.

14. Diczfalusy, E., Notter, G., Edsmyr, F., and Westman, A.: Estrogen excretion in breast cancer patients before and after ovarian irradiation and oophorectomy. J. Clin. Endocrinol., 19:1230–1244, 1959.

15. Kennedy, B. J., Mielke, P. W., Jr., and Fortuny, I. E.: Therapeutic castration versus prophylactic castration in breast cancer. Surg. Gynec. Obst., 118:524–540, 1964.

16. Nissen-Meyer, R.: Prophylactic endocrine treatment in carcinoma of the breast. Clin. Radiol., 15:152–160, 1964.

17. Dobson, L.: The management of metastatic breast cancer. Surg. Clin. N. Amer., 42:861–876, 1962.

18. Randall, H. T.: Oophorectomy and adrenalectomy in patients with inoperable or recurrent cancer of the breast. Amer. J. Surg., 99:553–561, 1960.

19. Huggins, C., and Bergenstal, D. M.: Inhibition of human mammary and prostatic cancers by adrenalectomy. Cancer Res., 12:134–141, 1952.

20. Dao, T. L., and Nemoto, T.: Evaluation of adrenalectomy and androgen in disseminated mammary carcinoma. Surg. Gynec. Obst., 121:1257–1262, 1965.

21. Deshpande, N., Bulbrook, R. D., and Ellis, F. G.: An apparent selective accumulation of testosterone by human breast tissue. J. Endocrinol., 25:555, 1963.

22. Vogler, W. R., Furtado, V. P., and Huguley, C. M., Jr.: Methotrexate for advanced cancer of the breast. Cancer, 21:26–30, 1968.

23. Nevinny, H. B., Hall, T. C., Haines, C., and Krant, M. J.: Comparison of methotrexate (NSC-740) and testosterone proprinate (NSC-9166) in the treatment of breast cancer. J. Clin. Pharm., 8:126–129, 1968.

24. Jacobs, E. M., Luce, J. K., and Wood, D. A.: Treatment of cancer with weekly intravenous 5-fluorouracil. Cancer, 22:1233–1238, 1968.

25. Mackman, S., Ramirez, G., and Ansfield, F. J.: Results of 5-fluorouracil (NSC-19893) given by the multiple daily dose method in disseminated breast cancer. Cancer Chemother. Rep., 51:483–489, 1967.

26. Jessiman, A. G., and Moore, F. D.: Carcinoma of the Breast: The Study and Treatment of the Patient. Boston, Little, Brown and Company, 1956.

27. Haddow, A., Watkinson, J. M., and Paterson, E.: Influence of synthetic oestrogens upon advanced malignant disease. Brit. Med. J., 2:393–398, 1944.
28. Talalay, P.: The scientific contributions of Charles Brenton Huggins. J.A.M.A., 192:1137–1140, 1965.
29. Jensen, E. V., DeSombre, E. R., and Jungblut, P. W.: Endogenous Factors Influencing Host-Tumor Balance. Chicago, University of Chicago Press, 1967, pp. 15–30.
30. Kleinfeld, G.: Acute fatal hypercalcemia: complication in estrogen therapy of metastatic breast cancer. J.A.M.A., 181:1137, 1962.
31. Kennedy, B. J.: Effect of massive doses of estradiol undecylate in advanced breast cancer. Cancer Chemother. Rep., 51:491–495, 1967.
32. Myers, W. P. L., West, C. D., Pearson, O. H., and Karnofsky, D. A.: Androgen-induced exacerbation of breast cancer measured by calcium excretion. Conversion of androgen to estrogen as a possible underlying mechanism. J.A.M.A., 161:127–131, 1956.
33. Muggia, F. M., et al.: Treatment of breast cancer with medroxyprogesterone acetate. Ann. Intern. Med., 68:328–337, 1968.
34. Crowley, L. G., and Macdonald, I.: Delalutin and estrogens for the treatment of advanced mammary carcinoma in the postmenopausal woman. Cancer, 18:436–446, 1965.
35. Holleb, A. I., Freeman, H. P., and Farrow, J. H.: Cancer of male breast. New York J. Med., 68:544–553 (Part I) and 656–663 (Part II), 1968.
36. Sandison, A. T.: Male breast cancer in Klinefelter's syndrome. Brit. J. Med., 1:521–522, 1965.
37. Treves, N.: The treatment of cancer, especially inoperable cancer of the male breast by ablative surgery (orchiectomy, adrenalectomy and hypophysectomy) and hormone therapy (estrogens and corticosteroids). An analysis of 42 patients. Cancer, 12:820, 1959.
38. Huggins, C., Jr., and Taylor, G. W.: Carcinoma of the male breast. Arch. Surg., 70:303–308, 1955.
39. Geller, J., Volk, H., and Lewin, M.: Objective remission of metastatic breast carcinoma in a male who received 17-alpha hydroxy progesterone caproate (Delalutin). Cancer Chemother. Rep., 14:77–81, 1961.

Additional Recent Bibliography Not Cited in the Text

40. Perlia, C. P., Gubisch, N. J., Wolter, J., Edelberg, D., Dederick, M. G., and Taylor, S. G., III: Mithramycin treatment of hypercalcemia. Cancer, 25:389–394, 1970.
41. Dodd, G. D., Wallace, J. D., Freundlich, I. M., Marsh, L., and Zermino, A.: Thermography and cancer of the breast. Cancer, 23:797–802, 1969.
42. Lemon, H. M.: Abnormal estrogen metabolism and tissue estrogen receptor proteins in breast cancer. Cancer, 25:423–435, 1970.

CHAPTER 5

MALIGNANT TUMORS OF THE GASTROINTESTINAL TRACT

CHEMOTHERAPY OF NONRESECTABLE PRIMARY AND METASTATIC NEOPLASMS

Surgery alone or in combination with radiation therapy is the primary modality of treatment of gastrointestinal neoplasms. Chemotherapy is reserved for the patient with a nonresectable primary lesion or disseminated disease. Combinations of chemotherapy and other modalities are also employed for management of disseminated disease.

Stomach

Gastric carcinoma is a disease of the fifth, sixth, and seventh decades of life. It is two or three times more common in men than in women.

For many years gastric carcinoma was one of the most frequent causes of cancer-related deaths in the United States. For unexplained reasons the incidence and the death rate from gastric cancer have decreased since the 1930's.[1] Carcinoma of the lung, skin, colon, and rectum is now more frequent than carcinoma of the stomach in males; carcinoma of the breast, uterus, and colon is more frequent in females.[2]

Carcinoma accounts for the great majority (about 90 per cent) of the malignant tumors of the stomach; lymphoma accounts for most of the remainder. Carcinoma spreads by local invasion and metastasis to the liver (49 per cent); peritoneum, omentum, and mesentery (43 per cent); lungs and pleura (33 per cent); ovary (14 per cent); and bone (11 per cent).[2] The reader is referred to the definitive work by

Stout[2] for a detailed discussion of the pathology of tumors of the stomach.

At present, the majority of patients with stomach cancer are not surgically curable at the time of diagnosis. Efforts to achieve earlier diagnosis for a larger segment of the population by means of various detection procedures applicable to screening large groups, for example, gastric cytology and fluoroscopic examination, have met with only limited success. Such procedures, including the gastrocamera, are more widely used in countries with a high incidence of gastric cancer, for example, Japan.

Colon and Rectum

Liechty et al.[3] recently reviewed the major clinical features of adenocarcinoma of the colon and rectum in 2261 patients over a 20-year period. Colorectal cancer accounts for 15 per cent of all cancer deaths in the United States and is surpassed in frequency only by carcinoma of the lung. The peak incidence occurs in the seventh decade of life, with equal frequency in males and in females. An important clinical observation is that between 50 and 75 per cent of colorectal tumors are within reach of the sigmoidoscope and therefore are diagnosable by a simple procedure.[3, 4] Pain and a change in bowel habits are the most common presenting symptoms of carcinoma of the colon and rectum.

Gross blood appears in the stools in 50 to 80 per cent of the patients with cancer of the rectum and left colon, but in only 30 per cent of those with cancer of the right colon.[4] Palpable masses at the time of diagnosis are much more common in right colonic lesions. The right colon has a wide lumen, so that symptoms of obstruction do not occur early in the disease. This fact may be reflected in the frequency with which right colonic lesions (as opposed to left-sided tumors) are found to be so far advanced as to preclude curative surgical resection.[4]

The mode of lymphatic spread of carcinoma of the colon is well understood.[5] A comprehensive treatment of the pathology of tumors of the intestinal tract is that by Wood.[6]

Liver, Biliary Tract, and Pancreas

In a series of 38 patients who had hepatic metastases from colonic and rectal carcinoma, 36 died within 12 months after diagnostic surgery.[7] The survival rates for primary malignant tumors of the liver are equally grim.[8] Edmondson[9] has written extensively on the pathology of primary hepatic tumors and has discussed the epidemiology. A common setting for the development of hepatoma is the liver already compromised by cirrhosis, either alcoholic or parasitic.

The results of treatment of carcinoma of the pancreas are also poor, and the 5-year survival rate is at best 5 to 10 per cent.[10]

A major problem in the clinical management of carcinoma of the pancreas is that the disease is almost always nonresectable at the time of diagnosis. This phenomenon reflects the facts that the carcinoma arises in a site that is not very accessible to the surgeon and that it grows in a silent fashion until the adjacent vital organs are invaded. There is at present no simple and reliable test for detection of early pancreatic carcinoma.

CHEMOTHERAPY PROGRAMS

It must be stated at the outset that chemotherapy benefits only a minority of patients with gastrointestinal carcinoma and is curative in none. The physician must weigh many factors before embarking on a course of chemotherapy—the patient's physical and psychologic ability to withstand a difficult and prolonged period of treatment, as well as social and financial factors. Because of the nature of the disease and the toxicities of the agents used in treatment, the physician must be prepared and have adequate facilities to monitor closely the changes occurring during the course of therapy. Despite these Cassandra-like warnings, it is clear that the picture is not nearly as gloomy now as it was even a few years ago. The introduction of 5-fluorouracil (5-FU) and the determination of the proper mode of its administration have added a whole new dimension to the picture. This compound is the cornerstone on which the chemotherapy of gastrointestinal cancer is built and its use will be considered in detail.

Although at present it is not clear that chemotherapeutic agents prolong the life of patients with disseminated gastrointestinal cancer, they often produce beneficial palliative effects, occasionally for 6 months or longer. In the chemotherapy of gastrointestinal carcinoma, as with other malignancies, objective criteria of tumor response should be used in assessing the effectiveness of the agent tried. These criteria include disappearance or reduction in the size of a palpable tumor, weight gain, improvement of liver function, and disappearance of abnormalities ascertained radiologically or by radioisotope scanning techniques. We have followed our patients with repeated tests of liver function (of which the alkaline phosphatase is usually most helpful) and by repeated radioisotopic scans of the liver.

There is sufficient clinical evidence to justify considering all the common gastrointestinal malignancies together in outlining a sequential scheme of chemotherapy.[11] For example, there is little differ-

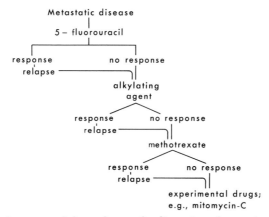

Figure 5–1   Sequence of chemotherapy for disseminated gastrointestinal cancer.

ence between the response rates of gastric and colorectal carcinoma to the most useful single agent, 5-FU. A suggested plan of sequential chemotherapy is shown in Figure 5–1. Not all patients can or should be treated according to this plan. It is also worth stressing that the usual 5-FU dosage may require modification for the poor-risk patient with colorectal cancer. (For example, see the four dosage schedules listed in Table 5–1.) Heidelberger and Ansfield[12] and Curreri et al.[13] have identified such poor-risk patients as those with cachexia, liver disease, and marrow infiltration, or patients previously treated with alkylating agents or pelvic irradiation, or both.

As indicated, the therapy of patients with disseminated gastrointestinal neoplasms improved considerably with the introduction of 5-FU.[12, 14] However, in view of the significant toxicity of 5-FU, this agent must still be viewed with tempered enthusiasm. It is now apparent that it can provide objective benefit to approximately 20 per cent of patients with nonresectable or metastatic gastrointestinal

TABLE 5–1   *Carcinoma of the Gastrointestinal Tract:*
5-Fluorouracil Dose Schedules

5-FLUOROURACIL LOADING DOSE	FOLLOW-UP DOSE	REFERENCE
1. 12 mg./kg./day x 4 or 5	6 mg./kg. every other day to toxicity	12
2. 5 mg./kg./day x 3	7.5 mg./kg. every other day to toxicity	20
3. 10 mg./kg./day x 3	7.5–10 mg./kg. every other day for at least 6 weeks or to toxicity	21
4. None	12.5–15 mg./kg. given once weekly until relapse or toxicity°	17

°In use at the University of California Hospitals, San Francisco.

neoplasms. With the introduction of modified programs of drug administration,[15-17] this benefit can now be achieved at an acceptably low level of drug toxicity. Although 5-FU is clearly the first line of defense in the management of the patient with disseminated gastrointestinal malignancy, this fact should not obscure earlier observations that some patients may be benefited by various alkylating agents or the antimetabolite, methotrexate. In the studies reported by the Eastern Solid Tumor Group for Colorectal Cancer,[18] the median duration of response to 5-FU was 11 weeks (range 3–42); for methotrexate, the median was 22 weeks (range 5–26 weeks). Patients responding to treatment lived longer than those who did not.

5-Fluorouracil is still relatively new, and the optimal dose schedule is still to be defined. It is clear that the initially described schedules had an unacceptably high morbidity and mortality (8 to 9 per cent) and that severe toxicity is not a necessary concomitant of tumor regression.[17, 19] In studies with more recently modified regimens, drug-induced mortality has been reduced to less than 2 per cent, and in some series it is nil.

It is worth reiterating the toxicities of 5-FU, since these are frequently used as guidelines to treatment. Bone marrow depression is the most serious complication. The white blood count usually falls somewhat before the platelet count, and maximal depression usually occurs within two weeks after the last dose. The white blood cell count should not be permitted to fall below 3000 per cu. mm. Diarrhea and stomatitis may also be serious complications of 5-FU treatment. The patient should not be treated to the point of severe stomatitis or bloody diarrhea. Nausea and anorexia are frequent complications of treatment. Alopecia may occur in as many as 25 per cent of treated patients, but it is usually reversible.[18]

Table 5–1 lists several modified dose schedules that have acceptable levels of toxicity and have produced regression rates of approximately 20 per cent.[12, 17, 20, 21] According to the program at the University of California Hospitals, San Francisco,[17] patients are given a test dose of 7.5 mg. per kg. and thereafter 15 mg. per kg. once weekly; after one month, the dose may be increased to 20 mg. per kg. once weekly if necessary. This program has been considered successful and produces only minimal toxicity. Treatment with 5-FU should be continued for at least 60 days before its efficacy is judged.

If a patient does not respond to 5-FU therapy or relapses after an initial response, alkylating agents and methotrexate may be considered for alternative therapy. These two classes of agents have comparable rates of induction of remission in colonic cancer. Several alkylating agents have been used with modest success, including chlorambucil, Thiotepa, and melphalan. Chlorambucil is the easiest to use and should be given orally in a dose of 0.1 mg. per kg. per day.

For rapid effects, nitrogen mustard, 0.4 mg. per kg., can be given intravenously.

The results with several methotrexate regimens have been reported. Perhaps the best results were obtained in a cooperative study in which methotrexate was given at a dose of 0.2 mg. per kg. for 4 days and then 0.1 mg. per kg. every other day until mild toxicity developed.[18] It is likely that this is not the optimal dose schedule and that even better results will be obtained with other schedules in the future.

Several agents that have undergone experimental clinical trials now appear promising in the treatment of certain gastrointestinal malignancies, for example, the antibiotic mitomycin-C.[22, 23]

Only recently has chemotherapy, alone or in combination with radiation therapy, been applied in a systematic way to malignant disease of the liver and pancreas. The results are still preliminary, and firm guidelines for chemotherapy have not been established. At least some patients with carcinoma of the pancreas appear to be benefited by chemotherapy in combination with radiation therapy.[10] In these lesions, the beneficial effect of 5-FU may last longer than 6 months.[24] Chlorambucil and other alkylating agents produce rare, good temporary results in cancer of this site and also in cancer of the liver and biliary tract.

The experience with small bowel neoplasms has been very limited because of the rarity of this tumor; however, the results with 5-FU seem comparable to those with other gastrointestinal neoplasms. Carcinoid tumors of the small intestine should be regarded as a distinct clinical entity and receive separate consideration (see Chapter 8).

COMBINATION OF CHEMOTHERAPY AND OTHER MODALITIES

A number of studies examining the question of whether combined radiation therapy and chemotherapy with 5-FU produces results superior to those with either modality alone have not been conclusive. A recent study by Childs and his collaborators[24] suggests that the results with radiation therapy plus 5-FU in adenocarcinoma of the stomach were superior to those with radiation therapy alone. In contrast, von Essen and his colleagues[25] found that the combination of radiation therapy and 5-FU in treating several types of tumors was not superior to the results with radiation therapy alone. In a well-analyzed study, Henderson et al.[26] concluded that "combination of 5-FU and ionizing radiation produces the same response as radiation alone, provided the radiation is given in sufficient amount. If not, the drug can act as a useful additive."

At the present time, it must be concluded that it is uncertain whether the combination of therapy with 5-FU and ionizing radiation is superior to optimally applied radiation alone. Similarly, there is no consensus as to the value of chemotherapy as a surgical adjuvant. A lack of certainty has been expressed about the usefulness of chemotherapy, for example, with 5-fluorodeoxyuridine (FUDR) as an adjuvant to primary surgical management of carcinoma of the stomach and colorectum.[27] Despite this generalization, it is clear that chemotherapy occasionally has place as an adjunct to surgery. In the same way that x-ray treatment is sometimes used to shrink a gastrointestinal tumor to a size that is manageable by the surgeon, chemotherapy (and in particular 5-FU) may rarely be used as an initial mode of attack before attempting surgical resection.

PERFUSION

Regional perfusion with chemotherapeutic agents must be considered as experimental, with no place as yet in established chemotherapeutic practice. A report of infusion of the liver with chemotherapeutic agents in cases of hepatic involvement by metastatic gastrointestinal malignancy aroused much interest,[28] but the results with this treatment in general have been disappointing.

It is my feeling that at the present time regional perfusion should be done in the limited number of institutions in which there is a particular interest in evaluating the effectiveness of this technique. Regional perfusion requires a dedicated team of surgeons working in close cooperation with medical oncologists. Because the potential complications of perfusion are many, it requires considerable experience to mount such a formidable attack on a noncurable malignancy. There is no place for such an attack at an institution that is not prepared to evaluate the results in a properly controlled fashion. This is not casual therapy to be undertaken by the amateur.

ILLUSTRATIVE CASE HISTORY: CARCINOMA OF THE APPENDIX

A 59-year-old man was in apparent good health until *March 1969*, when he "pulled his back." He stayed in bed one week because of severe low back pain with radiation to the hips and down both legs, and then returned to work. Three to 4 weeks later he noted difficulty in urination and developed urinary retention. An intravenous pyelogram showed obstruction of the neck of the bladder and a lesion of the L3 vertebra was noted, which was interpreted as an osteoblastic metastasis.

Carcinoma of the prostate was suspected; however, when a transurethral resection was performed, only benign prostatic tissue was found, and no evidence of malignancy. After roentgenologic studies of the gastrointestinal tract and a radioisotopic liver scan, the patient refused further studies and left the hospital against medical advice.

On *May 1, 1969*, the patient complained of a painful swelling in the right inguinal region and of nausea and vomiting. An exploratory laparotomy was performed and revealed adenocarcinoma of the appendix extending through the appendiceal wall and into the mesentery. A large "inflammatory mass" was removed.

After an uneventful 3-week postoperative period, the patient was referred to the University of California Hospitals, San Francisco. At that time he had severe back pain, anorexia, constipation, and weight loss. Physical examination (*July 5, 1969*) revealed a large irregular liver as well as a 5 cm. mass in the right lower quadrant. Spinal percussion tenderness as well as weakness and asymmetrical deep tendon reflexes of the lower extremities were noted.

Laboratory determinations included hematocrit of 36 per cent, positive tests for occult blood in the stool, and serum alkaline phosphatase of 298 IU per liter (normal, 25 to 80). A barium enema revealed a mass extrinsic to the cecum. A radioisotopic liver scan showed marked hepatomegaly with multifocal irregularities consistent with metastatic tumor. X-ray films of the spine showed metastases in the third and fifth lumbar vertebrae.

The plan of radiation therapy was to deliver 2500 to 3000 rads to the tumor in the area of the third lumbar vertebra. This course of therapy was started *July 17, 1969*.

Chemotherapy with 5-FU was begun *July 22, 1969*. The following tabulation summarizes the treatment and the patient's response:

DATE (1969)	5-FU DOSE (MG./WEEK)	WBC (COUNT/CU. MM.)	LIVER BELOW COSTAL MARGIN (CM.)	WEIGHT (KG.)	ALKALINE PHOSPHATASE (IU/LITER)
7/22	750 mg. × 1	7600	8	53	298
7/29	1000	8500	8–9	51.5	–
8/12	1000	6200	8	50	250
9/4	500	4400	6	51	180
9/11	750	4800	5–6	52	–
10/16	1000	5400	4	54	120
11/21	1000	5500	2–3	58	60

The patient's back pain and weakness of legs disappeared. Subsequently nausea and anorexia disappeared and the liver decreased in size. Studies of liver function also indicated improvement. The patient has gained weight and returned to work.

COMMENT: Metastatic disease from carcinoma of the appendix was managed with good response for 4 months with 5-FU and localized radiation therapy.

REFERENCES

1. Ackerman, L. V., and del Regato, J. A.: Cancer: Diagnosis, Treatment and Prognosis. Ed. 3. St. Louis, The C. V. Mosby Company, 1962, p. 580.
2. Stout, A. P.: Tumors of the stomach. In Atlas of Tumor Pathology. Washington, D.C., Armed Forces Institute of Pathology, 1953, Section VI, Fasc. 21.
3. Liechty, R. D., Ziffren, S. E., Miller, F. E., Coolidge, D., and DenBesten, L.: Adenocarcinoma of the colon and rectum: Review of 2,261 cases over a 20-year period. Dis. Colon Rectum, 11:201–208, 1968.
4. Bockus, H. L., Kalser, M. H., Mouhran, Y., Laucks, R., and Basset, J.: Early clinical manifestations of cancer of the colon and rectum. A statistical study. Dis. Colon Rectum, 2:58–68, 1959.
5. Gilchrist, R. K.: Lymphatic spread of carcinoma of the colon. Dis. Colon Rectum, 2:69–76, 1959.
6. Wood, D. A.: Tumors of the intestines. In Atlas of Tumor Pathology, Washington, D.C., Armed Forces Institute of Pathology, 1967, Section VI, Fasc. 22.
7. Bengmark, S., and Hafstrom, L.: The natural history of primary and secondary malignant tumors of the liver. Cancer, 23:198–202, 1969.
8. Phillips, R., and Murikami, K.: Primary neoplasms of the liver. Results of radiation therapy. Cancer, 13:714–720, 1960.
9. Edmondson, H. A.: Tumors of the liver and intrahepatic bile ducts. In Atlas of Tumor Pathology. Washington, D.C., Armed Forces Institute of Pathology, 1958, Section VII, Fasc. 25.
10. Gallitano, A., Fransen, H., and Martin, R. G.: Carcinoma of the pancreas. Results of treatment. Cancer, 22:939–944, 1968.
11. Schneiderman, M. A.: The clinical excursion into 5-fluorouracil. Cancer Chemother. Rep., 16:107, 1962.
12. Heidelberger, C., and Ansfield, F. J.: Experimental and clinical use of fluorinated pyrimidines in cancer chemotherapy. Cancer Res., 23:1226–1243, 1963.
13. Curreri, A. R., Ansfield, F. J., McIver, F. A., Waisman, H. A., and Heidelberger, C.: Clinical studies with 5-fluorouracil. Cancer Res., 18:478–484, 1958.
14. Heidelberger, C., et al.: Fluorinated pyrimidines, a new class of tumor-inhibitory compounds. Nature, 179:663–666, 1957.
15. Ansfield, F. J.: A less toxic fluorouracil dosage schedule. J.A.M.A., 190:686–688, 1964.
16. Moertel, C. G., and Reitemeier, R. J.: Chemotherapy of gastrointestinal cancer. Surg. Clin. N. Amer., 47:929, 1967.
17. Jacobs, E. M., Luce, J. K., and Wood, D. A.: Treatment of cancer with weekly intravenous 5-fluorouracil. Cancer, 22:1233–1238, 1968.
18. Hall, T. C.: A comparative study of 5-fluorouracil (FU), 5-fluorodeoxyuridine (FUDR) and methotrexate (MTX). Progress report. Cancer Chemother. Rep., 16:391, 1962.
19. Bross, I. D. J.: Is toxicity really necessary? (Abstract) Proc. Amer. Assoc. Cancer Res., 6:8, 1965.
20. A.M.A. Council on Drugs: New Drugs. Chicago, American Medical Association, 1965, p. 424.
21. Cudmore, J. T. P., and Groesbeck, H. P.: Comparison of high-dosage and low-dosage maintenance therapy with 5-fluorouracil in solid tumors. Cancer, 17:230–232, 1964.
22. Manheimer, L. H., and Vital, J.: Mitomycin-C in the therapy of far-advanced malignant tumors. Cancer, 19:207–212, 1966.
23. Moertel, C. G., Reitemeier, R. J., and Hahn, R. G.: Mitomycin C therapy in advanced gastrointestinal cancer. J.A.M.A., 204:1045–1048, 1968.
24. Childs, D. S., Jr., Moertel, C. G., Holbrook, M. A., Reitemeier, R. J., and Colby, M., Jr.: Treatment of unresectable adenocarcinomas of the stomach with a combination of 5-fluorouracil and radiation. Amer. J. Roent., 102:541–544, 1968.
25. von Essen, C. F., Kligerman, M. M., and Calabresi, P.: Radiation and 5-fluorouracil: A controlled clinical study. Radiology, 81:1018–1027, 1963.

26. Henderson, I. W. D., Lipowska, B., Lougheed, S. I., and Lougheed, M. N.: Clinical evaluation of combined radiation and chemotherapy in gastrointestinal malignancies. Amer. J. Roent., 102:545–551, 1968.
27. Higgins, G. A., Jr. (Veterans Administration Adjuvant Cancer Chemotherapy Cooperative Group): The use of 5-fluorodeoxyuridine (FUDR) as a surgical adjuvant in carcinoma of the stomach and colorectum. Arch. Surg., 86:926–931, 1963.
28. Sullivan, R. D., Norcross, J. W., and Watkins, E., Jr.: Chemotherapy of metastatic liver cancer by prolonged hepatic-artery infusion. New Eng. J. Med., 270:321–327, 1964.

CHAPTER 6

CARCINOMA OF THE LUNG

The survival rate of patients with inoperable carcinoma of the lung is very low indeed. In the majority of patients with nonresectable or recurrent pulmonary cancer, it is not possible to achieve more than short-term palliation by radiation therapy. There is considerable doubt whether radiation therapy increases the rate of survival beyond that achieved by optimal medical management alone.[1-3] Caldwell and Bagshaw[1] note that "No pretreatment criteria allow the radiotherapist categorically to decide definitively which patients might be cured and which might receive palliation only." It appears unlikely that nitrogen mustard, actinomycin-D, or 5-FU used in combination with radiation therapy is superior to radiation therapy alone.[4-6]

In view of these considerations, is there any place for established (as opposed to experimental) chemotherapy in treating the patient with nonresectable carcinoma of the lung at the present time? It is impossible to give a categorical answer to this question. One must review the objectives of using chemotherapeutic agents: to prolong survival or reduce morbidity, or both. Reducing tumor size by 25 to 50 per cent without any associated objective benefit to the patient is not a sufficiently good criterion for drug administration. If one reviews the literature with regard to nonresectable lung tumors, one finds that prolongation of mean survival has not been achieved by means of any agent or combination of agents. Reduction of the size of the pulmonary tumor may be observed after treatment with a number of drugs, including various alkylating agents, procarbazine, and methotrexate,[6-9] but often the patient's condition continues to deteriorate although his tumor is smaller.[10] Despite the generally gloomy picture, occasional patients appear to be unequivocally benefited by chemotherapeutic drugs. It is not possible to give a firm

88

estimate of the percentage of patients with carcinoma of the lung who will obtain such benefit, but it is probably less than 10 per cent.

In view of these considerations, the policy recommended here is to administer alkylating agents when the patient can tolerate them without undue risk or inconvenience. If the patient is ambulatory, an alkylating agent such as chlorambucil is given by mouth in doses of 4 to 6 mg. per day. If a rapid therapeutic trial is indicated, nitrogen mustard, 0.4 or 0.5 mg. per kg., may be given intravenously.

Recurrent pleural effusions are often controlled by means of chemotherapy. A plan of sequential therapy is presented and discussed in Chapter 14.

It is only fair to point out that some chemotherapists take a much more aggressive approach to the treatment of nonresectable carcinoma of the lung.[11] Clearly, a new therapeutic approach is needed. Bronchial artery infusion of chemotherapeutic agents may be one such approach.[12]

A number of endocrinologic syndromes have been reported with lung tumors. The most common are Cushing's syndrome secondary to carcinoma that secretes corticotropin-like polypeptides[13] and carcinoma with inappropriate antidiuretic hormone secretion.[14] In addition, bronchial carcinoid tumors may produce other pharmacologically active substances (see Chapter 8). The most common hormonally active lung tumor is oat cell carcinoma, but bronchial adenoma may also be active.[15] Such hormonal irregularities are grafted to the already complex problem of a malignant disease. Careful medical management is required and sometimes pharmacologic treatment of the hormonal syndrome is necessary, as described in Chapter 8.

REFERENCES

1. Caldwell, W. L., and Bagshaw, M. A.: Indications for and results of irradiation of carcinoma of the lung. Cancer, 22:999–1004, 1968.
2. Wolf, J.: Controlled studies of the therapy of nonresectable cancer of the lung. I. Methodology. Ann. Thorac. Surg., 1:25–32, 1965.
3. Wolf, J., Patno, M. E., Roswit, B., and D'Esopo, N.: Controlled study of survival of patients with clinically inoperable lung cancer treated with radiation therapy. Amer. J. Med., 40:360–367, 1966.
4. Chalmers, T. C.: Combination of radiotherapy and chemotherapy in the treatment of carcinoma of the lung. Cancer Chemother. Rep., 16:463, 1962.
5. Krant, M. J., et al.: Comparative trial of chemotherapy and radiotherapy in patients with non-resectable cancer of the lung. Amer. J. Med., 35:363–373, 1963.
6. Hall, T. C., et al.: A clinical pharmacologic study of chemotherapy and x-ray therapy in lung cancer. Amer. J. Med., 43:186–193, 1967.
7. Ross, C. A., and Selawry, O. S.: Comparison of three dosage schedules of methotrexate in lung cancer. (Abstract) Proc. Amer. Assoc. Cancer Res., 6:54, 1965.
8. De La Garza, J. G., Carr, D. T., and Bisel, H. F.: Hexamethylmelamine (NSC-13875) in the treatment of primary cancer of the lung with metastasis. Cancer, 22:571–575, 1968.
9. Samuels, M. L., Leary, W. V., and Howe, C. D.: Procarbazine (NSC-77213) in the

treatment of advanced bronchogenic carcinoma. Cancer Chemother. Rep., 53:135, 1969.

10. Reed, L. J., Muggia, F. M., Klipstein, F. A., and Gellhorn, A.: Intermittent parenteral methotrexate (NSC-740) therapy for carcinoma of the lung. Cancer Chemother. Rep., 51:475–481, 1967.

11. Weiss, A. J.: Chemotherapy of lung cancer. *In* Brodsky, I., Kahn, S. B., and Moyer, J. H. (Editors): Cancer Chemotherapy. New York, Grune & Stratton, Inc., 1967, p. 148.

12. Neyazaki, T., Ikeda, M., Seki, Y., Egawa, N., and Suzuki, C.: Bronchial artery infusion therapy for lung cancer. Cancer, 24:912–922, 1969.

13. O'Riordan, J. L. H., Blanchard, G. P., Moxham, A., and Nabarro, J. D. N.: Corticotrophin-secreting carcinomas. Quart. J. Med., 35:137–147, 1966.

14. Sawyer, W. H.: Pharmacological characteristics of the antidiuretic principle in a bronchogenic carcinoma from a patient with hyponatremia. J. Clin. Endocrinol. Metab., 27:497–1499, 1967.

15. Strott, C. A., Nugent, C. A., and Tyler, F. H.: Cushing's syndrome caused by bronchial adenomas. Amer. J. Med., 44:97–104, 1968.

Additional Recent Bibliography Not Cited in Text

16. Kato, Y., Ferguson, T. B., Bennett, D. E., and Burford, T. H.: Oat cell carcinoma of the lung. A review of 138 cases. Cancer, 23:517–524, 1969.

17. Slack, N. H.: Bronchogenic carcinoma: Nitrogen mustard as a surgical adjuvant and factors influencing survival. University surgical adjuvant lung project. Cancer, 25:987–1002, 1970.

18. Cliffton, E. E.: Bronchial artery perfusion for treatment of advanced lung cancer. Cancer, 23:1151–1157, 1969.

CHAPTER 7

CANCER OF THE HEAD AND NECK

CLASSIFICATION AND PROGNOSIS

In the context of this chapter, cancer of the head and neck includes tumors arising from nasopharyngeal, hypopharyngeal, and oropharyngeal tissues, from the paranasal sinuses, and from the salivary glands. A variety of histologic types of tumors are represented. There is no uniform agreement as to their histogenesis or pathologic classification. A classification of malignant tumors of the pharynx and nasopharynx follows.[1, 2]

Epithelial
> Squamous cell (well-differentiated, transitional cell, anaplastic)
> Lymphoepithelioma
> Adenocarcinoma (rare)

Nonepithelial
> Lymphomas
> Plasmacytoma (rare)
> Fibrosarcoma (rare)

Although there is controversy as to whether lymphoepithelioma should be included in the group of tumors that are primarily of epithelial origin, there are good clinical reasons for doing so.

By far the most common malignant tumors of the pharynx and sinuses are of epithelial origin. These tumors spread by local invasion and lymph node metastasis. The pattern of spread to regional lymphatics has been reviewed recently.[1, 2]

Certain features of these epithelial tumors are worth reviewing briefly. The prognosis is a function of the extent of spread (stage) of

91

the tumor and, to a lesser extent, of the histologic type. The 5-year survival rate varies from 46 per cent in patients with no clinically palpable nodes to only 7 per cent in those with fixed nodes. Survival is somewhat better in women than in men and is somewhat poorer in orientals than in Caucasians. Lymphoepithelioma has a somewhat better prognosis than squamous cell carcinoma. Bone erosion at the base of the skull or intracranial extension and cranial nerve involvement are equivalent to distant metastasis and have a poor prognosis. The neurologic manifestations of nasopharyngeal tumors have been reviewed recently.[3]

THERAPY

Central to the management of cancers of the head and neck is the concept that the primary modalities of definitive therapy with curative intent are radiation therapy and surgery. The primary mode of attack on nasopharyngeal tumors is radiation therapy;[1, 2] on malignancies of salivary gland origin, it is surgery.[4–6]

The radiosensitivity of malignant tumors of epithelial origin cannot be predicted from histologic appearance alone, but must be determined by clinical trial. In general, lymphoepithelioma and transitional cell carcinoma are considered to be radiosensitive.

Malignant lymphoma arising in the head and neck is staged in the same manner as lymphoma arising in other sites (see Chapter 12). The general principles for the treatment of lymphoma are also applicable to lymphoma arising in the pharynx. Waldeyer's ring is a frequent site of origin of lymphoma of the head and neck. The anatomy of this region is such as to place certain restrictions on the radiotherapist.[1, 2]

Several reviews of tumors originating in the salivary glands have appeared recently that include a discussion of the complex pathology as well as the natural history and approach to the management of salivary gland malignancies.[4–6] A large series of cases of carcinoma of the buccal mucosa, palate, and gingiva has also been reported recently.[7]

Chemotherapy

Chemotherapy is reserved for the tumor that is no longer amenable to surgery or radiation therapy. Rarely chemotherapy is used to shrink a very large tumor prior to the institution of radiation therapy.

Whether chemotherapy should ever be used for cancer of salivary gland origin is open to question. There is definitely a place for chemotherapy, however, in the management of advanced pharyngeal malignancies of epithelial origin.

According to most recent reports, approximately 50 per cent of the patients with cancer of the head and neck have benefited from cytotoxic drugs. The most commonly used single agent has been methotrexate. The recent trend has been to treat patients with large doses of methotrexate in weekly courses rather than with small daily oral doses. A summary of several recently reported dose schedules is given in Table 7-1.[8-10]

Preliminary evidence indicates that some chemotherapeutic drugs in combination with radiation therapy may be useful in the treatment of far-advanced epidermoid carcinoma of the buccal mucosa. More data are necessary, however, before such combinations can be considered "standard."

Occasionally patients with carcinoma of the head and neck who fail to respond to methotrexate or who relapse after initially responding may be benefited by alkylating agents. It is difficult to ascertain the precise percentage of responsive patients, but it is probably less than 15 per cent. Remissions with alkylating agents are generally of short duration.

PERFUSION. Local perfusion with chemotherapeutic agents has been used alone or in conjunction with radiation therapy in the treatment of head and neck cancer.[11, 12] Such therapy is still experimental. Although it is efficacious in some patients, it is a difficult and at times dangerous procedure. Jesse and his colleagues[12] reported a study in which 46 patients with advanced cancer of the head and neck were treated with intra-arterial methotrexate or 5-FU combined with radiation therapy. Infusions were given in two 5-day courses and a total of 6000 to 7000 rads was given over a 6- to 7-week period. Therapy was not completed in 12 of the 46 patients because of "severe local toxicity, distant metastases appearing during therapy, or the patient's desire to stop treatment." Of the remaining patients, 12 were classified as failures, 10 developed local recurrence of disease, and 12 (approximately one-fourth of the original series) were apparently free of local disease 8 to 60 months after therapy. However, only 5 of these 12 were living and well; the rest had died of the original or other malignancy.

TABLE 7-1 *Methotrexate Therapy for Cancer of the Head and Neck*

DOSE SCHEDULE	BENEFICIAL RESPONSES	COMPLETE REGRESSIONS	SEVERE TOXICITY	REFERENCE
20–50 mg. I.V. every 4–7 days	14/27	4/27	6/27	8
1–3 mg./kg. over 24 hours; leucovorin given°	4/18	>75% regression in 3/18	dose-dependent	9
60 mg./sq. M./week	20/35	11/35	3/35 died	10

°Experimental.

Toxicity associated with this program was of variable severity. With methotrexate there was "usually moderate local toxicity" and systemic toxicity with leukopenia and thrombocytopenia. 5-FU produced local toxicity, with erythema progressing to patchy ulceration of skin and mucosa. Moist desquamation and necrosis of the external ear were occasionally seen. At the moment one must ask whether the modest results achieved by this therapy were worth the effort. The results do not seem to be clearly superior to those achieved by radiation therapy alone.

Perfusion techniques should be reserved for experimental cancer treatment centers. If they are employed, a skilled chemotherapist must work in concert with a skilled surgeon who has managed many such cases.

ILLUSTRATIVE CASE HISTORY: SQUAMOUS CELL CARCINOMA OF THE TONGUE AND FLOOR OF THE MOUTH

A 51-year-old man with a history of alcoholism first noted a painful lesion on the anterior tongue in *December 1960*. Nine months later the lesion had grown so much that the patient had difficulty in eating and talking. A biopsy revealed squamous cell carcinoma. In *November 1961*, the patient was seen by the Consultative Tumor Board at the University of California Hospitals, San Francisco. Because difficulty in resection was anticipated, radiation therapy was advised.

The patient was treated on an experimental protocol combining radiation therapy and 5-FU, beginning in early *December 1961*. There was slight but definite objective improvement in the lesion over a 6-week period. However, by mid-*January 1962*, metastatic masses were found in the neck (Fig. 7–1A), and the first of several episodes of oral hemorrhage occurred.

In *February 1962*, treatment with methotrexate was begun. It was given intravenously in monthly courses of 25 mg. on each of 4 or 5 days. The dose was adjusted downward when the patient developed transient leukopenia. No other symptoms of drug toxicity were noted. Over the course of several months there was subjective improvement in swallowing and decreased pain; there was also an objective response, shown by reduction in the size of metastatic lesions (Fig. 7–1B and C). Seven months after initiation of therapy only a small ulcer of the posterior right mandible and small cervical nodes remained. At that time the patient went on an alcoholic binge and was lost to further follow-up care. It was subsequently learned that he had died in *January 1963*. The masses in the neck and oral cavity had enlarged and then bled massively. The patient was thought to have had terminal aspiration pneumonia.

COMMENT: This case illustrates the benefit that may occasionally be achieved by intensive treatment of squamous cell carcinoma of the head and neck with methotrexate.

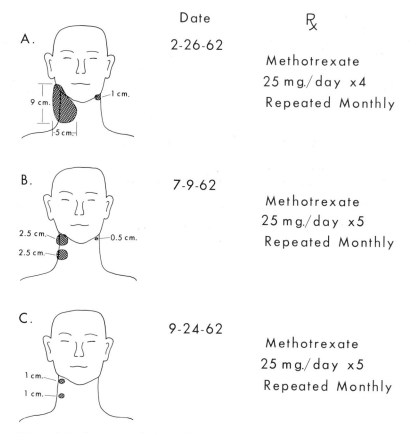

Figure 7–1 Sequence of chemotherapy and tumor response in a patient with squamous cell carcinoma of the tongue.

REFERENCES

1. Lederman, M.: Cancer of the pharynx. J. Laryng. Otol., *81*:151, 1967.
2. Fletcher, G. H., and Million, R. R.: Malignant tumors of the nasopharynx. Amer. J. Roent., *93*:44–55, 1965.
3. Thomas, J. E., and Waltz, A. G.: Neurological manifestations of nasopharyngeal malignant tumors. J.A.M.A., *192*:95–98, 1965.
4. Morgan, M. N., and Mackenzie, D. H.: Tumours of salivary glands. A review of 204 cases with 5-year follow-up. Brit. J. Surg., *55*:284–288, 1968.
5. Bardwil, J. M.: Tumors of the parotid gland. Amer. J. Surg., *114*:498–502, 1967.
6. Rosenfeld, L., Sessions, D., McSwain, B., and Graves, H.: Malignant tumors of salivary gland origin: 37-year review of 184 cases. Ann. Surg. *163*:726–735, 1966.
7. Shedd, D. P., von Essen, C. F., Connelly, R. R., and Eisenberg, H.: Cancer of the buccal mucosa, palate and gingiva in Connecticut, 1935–1959. Cancer, *21*:440–446, 1968.
8. Lane, M., Moore, J. E., III, Levin, H., and Smith, F. E.: Methotrexate therapy for squamous cell carcinomas of the head and neck. J.A.M.A., *204*:561–564, 1968.
9. Lefkowitz, E., Papac, R. J., and Bertino, J. R.: Head and neck cancer. III. Toxicity of 24-hour infusions of methotrexate (NSC-740) and protection by leucovorin

(NSC-3590) in patients with epidermoid carcinomas. Cancer Chemother. Rep., 51:305–311, 1967.

10. Leone, L. A., Albala, M. M., and Rege, V. B.: Treatment of carcinoma of the head and neck with intravenous methotrexate. Cancer, 21:828–837, 1968.

11. Lawrence, W., Jr.: Current status of regional chemotherapy. New York State J. Med., 63:2359–2382 (Part I: Technics) and 2518–2534 (Part II: Results), 1963.

12. Jesse, R. H., Goepfert, H., Lindberg, R. D., and Johnson, R. H.: Combined intra-arterial infusion and radiotherapy for the treatment of advanced cancer of the head and neck. Amer. J. Roent., 105:20–25, 1969.

Additional Recent Bibliography Not Cited in Text

13. Schnohr, P.: Survival rates of nasopharyngeal cancer in California: A review of 516 cases from 1942 through 1965. Cancer, 25:1099–1106, 1970.

14. Ansfield, F. J., Ramirez, G., Davis, H. L., Jr., Korbitz, B. C., Vermund, H., and Gollin, F. F.: Treatment of advanced cancer of the head and neck. Cancer, 25:78–82, 1970.

15. Lund, W. S.: The external carotid artery (a perfusion technique used in 30 patients with head and neck cancer). J. Laryng. Otol., 83:609–612, 1969.

CHAPTER 8

ENDOCRINE TUMORS

Certain malignant endocrine tumors are of particular interest to the medical oncologist. The clinical manifestations of these tumors are often a function of both the malignant process and biologically active tumor products. The therapeutic approach to such endocrinologically active tumors must necessarily involve not only procedures directed against the malignancy but also the control or inhibition of the excess hormones or other substances the tumors produce.

PHEOCHROMOCYTOMA

Pheochromocytoma, although rare, is the most important hormonally active tumor of the adrenal medulla. The current concepts of diagnosis and treatment of malignant pheochromocytoma have been reviewed recently.[1] Certain clinical manifestations of this disease syndrome bear emphasis. In addition to paroxysmal hypertension, excessive perspiration or an orthostatic decrease in blood pressure in an untreated patient are important clues to the diagnosis of pheochromocytoma.[2] The diagnosis of a neuroectodermal disease such as von Recklinghausen's neurofibromatosis or von Hippel-Lindau disease should arouse suspicion of the possibility of a pheochromocytoma. Similarly, the occurrence of hyperparathyroidism or medullary thyroid carcinoma should always suggest adrenal pheochromocytoma as part of a clinical triad.[3]

The definitive treatment for pheochromocytoma is surgery; however, approximately 5 per cent of the patients have metastatic malignancy not amenable to surgical management. For patients with disseminated disease, the therapeutic alternatives are chemotherapy or pharmacologic blockade of the tumor products. In view of the poor results presently obtainable with cytotoxic drugs, medical management is to be preferred. Such management can ameliorate symptoms and prolong life. At the present time, the use of cytotoxic chemotherapeutic agents is not recommended for the treatment of malignant pheochromocytoma.

Therapy is based on the principle that the patient with malignant pheochromocytoma is likely to die of uncontrolled cardiovascular changes related to catecholamine production long before the slowly growing tumor is itself fatal.

At the present time, the drug of choice for treating the patient who is not a candidate for operation is an alpha-adrenergic blocking agent such as phenoxybenzamine (Dibenzyline).[4] Such agents block the pharmacologic effects of catecholamines produced by the tumor. The use of inhibitors of catecholamine synthesis (as opposed to adrenergic blocking agents) is still experimental and is not recommended.

Control of symptomatic malignant pheochromocytoma with alpha-adrenergic blocking agents can be continued for several years.[4] Phenoxybenzamine, given orally in divided doses (usually every 8 to 12 hours) totaling 40 to 100 mg. daily, is usually sufficient to control blood pressure, hypertensive attacks, and other symptoms such as sweating.

Phentolamine (Regitine) is generally unsatisfactory for long-term treatment but is often effective for rapid and short-term control of blood pressure. Hydralazine and reserpine are inadequate for controlling the manifestations of increased catecholamine production and, in fact, may be dangerous. Although guanethidine has occasionally been used for long-term treatment,[5] this drug should be used with caution in the patient with pheochromocytoma because of its ability to release pharmacologically active tumor products.

CARCINOID TUMORS

The metabolic derangements and clinical manifestations of carcinoid tumors are complex and fascinating.[6, 7] Since these manifestations vary with the primary site of the tumor, it is appropriate to consider a carcinoid spectrum rather than a single syndrome.[7] The classic syndrome occurs in association with a primary tumor in the small intestine. Variants of the syndrome are observed with gastric carcinoid and bronchial carcinoid tumors. Because of their rich variety of pharmacologically active products, these tumors have been studied primarily by clinical pharmacologists rather than by oncologists. Consequently, considerable attention has been focused on the biochemical pathways involved in the synthesis of biologically active compounds by the tumor, and relatively little attention has been devoted to the "total therapy of this disease."[8]

Surgery

Whenever possible, *the initial therapeutic attack should be surgical removal of the primary tumor,* which is usually in the small intestine,[9] sometimes in the lung[10] or stomach,[11] and occasionally in other sites.[8] Unfortunately, the diagnosis is seldom made before metastasis has occurred. The decision to perform surgery in the patient with carcinoid syndrome cannot be made casually. Patients with this disease are sensitive to a variety of anesthetic agents, which may precipitate severe hypotension and bronchial constriction. Frequent complications of surgery are adhesions and subsequent bowel obstruction.[8]

Surgery is not limited to resection of the primary lesion. For example, removal of large isolated metastatic lesions of the liver or omentum may ameliorate the disease by removing a major source of production of serotonin and vasoactive peptides.[12, 13] Mengel[8] has suggested that preoperative analysis of the serotonin content of blood samples from the left and right hepatic veins may be useful in making a decision regarding hepatic surgery. Surgery of metastatic lesions may also apply to bronchial carcinoid tumors.[14]

Radiation Therapy

Carcinoid tumors are generally resistant to radiation therapy, although sporadic reports of good responses exist in the literature.[15]

Chemotherapy

There is no consistent evidence that chemotherapy prolongs the life of the patient with carcinoid tumor or even reduces morbidity. Therefore, all chemotherapy in this disease syndrome should still be considered experimental. No well-organized body of information exists in the literature regarding the optimal chemotherapeutic approach. Reports of chemotherapeutic trials are fragmentary and difficult to evaluate. Both nitrogen mustard and 5-FU have been tried, with occasional good responses.[16, 17] Hepatic artery perfusion with 5-FU has been tried with modest success.[18] Methotrexate in large weekly doses appeared to benefit one patient.[8] In another study, hepatic tumors regressed by 25 per cent or more in four of eight patients treated with cyclophosphamide,[8] but these patients received no real benefit from the drug. In fact, exacerbations of symptoms occurred during the cyclophosphamide treatment, presumably as a result of tumor cell destruction and release of active compounds.

It would appear that if chemotherapy is used at all, serotonin or histamine antagonists should be used simultaneously if symptoms of these pharmacologically active amines appear or increase in intensity.

Control of Pharmacologically Active Products

Antagonists of pharmacologically active tumor products are useful drugs in the treatment of carcinoid tumors. These tumors elaborate a number of pharmacologically active compounds, including a host of tryptophan metabolites and biologically active peptides such as bradykinin.[6] Serotonin production may be related to gastrointestinal symptoms, but has an inconstant association with flushing; flushing may be related to elaboration of vasoactive polypeptides such as kinins.[12]

If gastrointestinal symptoms are a major problem, and if the 5-hydroxyindoleacetic acid (5-HIAA) excretion is high, then serotonin antagonists may be useful in producing symptomatic relief. Serotonin antagonists are generally not useful for relief of flushing or bronchial constriction and apparently do not affect the development of cardiac lesions. They may, however, relieve abdominal cramps, diarrhea, and even reverse steatorrhea.[19] In general, however, symptomatic management of the gastrointestinal symptoms suffices.

Several approaches to reducing the effects of serotonin have been tried. Interference with serotonin synthesis by the induction of tryptophan or vitamin B_6 deficiency apparently is not clinically useful. Inhibition of serotonin synthesis by enzymatic inhibitors of 5-hydroxytryptophan decarboxylase[8] or of hydroxylation of tryptophan[20] are experimental procedures that are unlikely to be generally useful clinically. At the present time, serotonin antagonists are the most effective pharmacologic agents for treating the patient with severe abdominal symptoms. These drugs include methysergide (Sansert) and cyproheptadine (Periactin). Methysergide must be used cautiously; its prolonged administration tends to produce retroperitoneal fibrosis. In addition, the serotonin antagonists may cause weakness, lassitude, hypotension, and syncope. Methysergide maleate should be used intermittently during symptomatic periods in doses of 8 to 32 mg. during a 24-hour period. The dosage should be scheduled to correspond to peak symptomatic periods. Therapy should be interrupted periodically to prevent or delay the emergence of drug resistance.[8] It must be stressed that the response to this agent is not predictable. It is only occasionally effective in controlling flushing.

Phenothiazine drugs may often be useful in controlling flushing[6, 10] but not always.[8] No clinically effective antikinin agents are known.[21] Adrenocorticosteroids appear to be of benefit for symptomatic relief of patients with bronchial carcinoid tumors. In occasion-

TABLE 8-1 *Medical Management of Carcinoid Syndromes*

SYNDROME	MANIFESTATION	PHARMACOLOGIC MEDIATOR	TREATMENT
Small bowel and hepatic carcinoid	G.I. disturbance: diarrhea, cramps, malabsorption	? Serotonin and metabolites	Antispasmodics, anticholinergics Serotonin antagonists: methysergide, cyproheptadine
All carcinoid syndromes	Flushing	? Kinins	Phenazine drugs, e.g., prochlorperazine, promazine
Especially bronchial carcinoid	Bronchospasm	? Kinins	Adrenocorticosteroids; hydrocortisone, prednisolone for rapid effect

al patients with life-threatening manifestations of bronchial carcinoid tumors, adrenal steroids in high dosage may be life-saving.

The medical management of the manifestations of the carcinoid syndromes is summarized in Table 8-1.

ILLUSTRATIVE CASE HISTORY: CARCINOID TUMOR

The clinical course of this patient's illness and his response to therapy are illustrated in Figure 8-1.

The patient first noted the onset of frequent diarrhea in 1961 at the age of 42. About 1 year later intermittent cramping and epigastric pain occurred. These symptoms were attributed to a stressful work situation as an electronics engineer. Antacids and antispasmodics provided some relief of pain and diarrhea. The patient developed severe right upper quadrant pain in 1964.

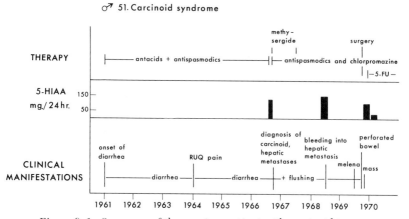

Figure 8-1 Sequence of therapy in a patient with carcinoid tumor.

The findings of an upper gastrointestinal series, barium enema studies, and sigmoidoscopy were normal, and his complaints were considered to be of a functional nature. Symptomatic relief of diarrhea was achieved with Lomotil.

It was not until the finding of an elevated urinary 5-hydroxy-indolacetic acid (5-HIAA) level in *August 1966* that the diagnosis of carcinoid syndrome was suspected and the patient was referred to the University of California Hospitals, San Francisco.

The findings of physical examination were normal except for the patient's slightly plethoric appearance. No hepatomegaly was detectable. Results of laboratory studies including tests for malabsorption, serum electrolytes, and serum alkaline phosphatase were within normal ranges. No definite abnormalities were detectable by means of a roentgenographic survey of the gastrointestinal tract. However, percutaneous biopsy of the liver revealed microscopic foci of tumor cells consistent with carcinoid tumor, and the 24-hour urine excretion of 5-HIAA was 144 mg. (normal, 1 to 9 mg.). Before discharge from the hospital, the patient received a brief trial of methysergide, a serotonin antagonist, in 2 mg. doses given 4 times daily. This therapy resulted in a decrease in frequency of bowel movements (to one per day). When the patient left the hospital late in *November 1966*, he was taking the following medications: methysergide, 8 mg. daily; chlorpromazine, 100 mg. daily in divided doses; and deodorized tincture of opium (DTO), 6 drops twice daily. On this program, stools were only slightly less frequent. Therefore, in *July 1967*, the methysergide was discontinued and the only medications were an antispasmodic and chlorpromazine.

On *July 25, 1968*, the patient consulted his physician because of dull aching upper abdominal pain of one week's duration. The edge of the liver was felt 2 fingerbreadths below the costal margin, and a round mass was palpable in the region posterior and inferior to the liver's edge. This mass had not been noted previously. In *August 1966*, when the patient entered the University of California Hospitals, San Francisco, for the second time, he was having 8 to 10 watery stools daily. Another symptom was frequent flushing, which, however, caused him no discomfort. He had lost 10 pounds in weight over a 3-month period and had recurrence of the right upper quadrant pain. A radioisotopic liver scan demonstrated slight hepatomegaly and several discrete defects consistent with metastatic disease. His physicians felt that the clinical picture was most consistent with a recent hemorrhage into a metastatic lesion of the liver. The patient left the hospital on *August 8, 1968*, on a program of restricted activity. The abdominal pain and the hepatic mass gradually disappeared.

His clinical condition remained unchanged until *June 1969*, when he was re-evaluated because of melena and transient symptoms of partial bowel obstruction. A barium enema revealed a right lower quadrant mass. He was given only symptomatic therapy for the next 4 months. In *October 1969*, an acute abdominal emergency necessitated a laparotomy, and perforation of a carcinoid tumor of the ileum was found as well as a metastatic hepatic tumor. An ileotransverse colostomy was performed. An enterocutaneous fistula was a complication of his tumor and surgery. Because of intractable diarrhea, anorexia, and weight loss of 25 pounds, the patient re-entered the hospital for the third time in *December 1969* to be evaluated for experimental chemotherapy.

A new 8 by 10 cm. hard mass was palpable in the right upper quadrant. Low serum calcium, elevated serum alkaline phosphatase, and increased fecal fat excretion were found. The patient was placed on a regimen consisting of deodorized tincture of opium, chlorpromazine, and a diet containing medium-chain triglycerides, low in theophylline and serotonin. There was a slight decrease in the frequency of stools as a result of this program.

A series of quantitative determinations of urinary excretion of 5-HIAA were made before an experimental program of 5-fluorouracil was begun on December 20, 1969. 5-FU was given in weekly doses of 500 to 750 mg. and the peripheral white blood count, the urinary 5-HIAA level, and the size of the abdominal mass were closely monitored. By *February 3, 1970*, the patient felt well although the mass had increased in size to 10 by 11 cm. and the diarrhea was unchanged. The 24-hour urinary 5-HIAA excretion had decreased from a pretreatment value in the range 100 to 110 mg. to 35 mg.

By *March 3, 1970*, the frequency of bowel movements had decreased to 5 or 6 per day, and a decrease in the size of the mass to 6 by 10 cm. was noted. The situation was unchanged late in March, 1970.

COMMENT: For many years the patient's abdominal symptoms were treated with antispasmodics, phenathiazines, and a brief course of methysergide. Laparotomy was delayed until an acute abdominal crisis forced surgical intervention. Nine years after the onset of symptoms, when the patient's condition was such that he no longer responded to conservative treatment, chemotherapy with an experimental agent was instituted. After 5 months of such 5-FU therapy, there was no definite improvement in the patient's condition, although the rate of excretion of 5-HIAA diminished.

CARCINOMA OF THE ADRENAL CORTEX

Adrenocortical carcinoma is rare. This malignancy tends to occur in young individuals and carries a very poor prognosis. Of 38 patients in a series reported by the National Cancer Institute, half were dead within two years.[22] This tumor presents the difficult problem of a rapidly advancing malignancy combined with the flagrant clinical manifestations of Cushing's syndrome. In general, adrenal carcinoma produces large quantities of steroids (>100 mg. of 17-ketosteroids and 50 mg. of 11-hydroxysteroids in 24 hours). The associated electrolyte imbalance and abnormalities of carbohydrate metabolism are often profound.

The primary therapeutic attack on malignant tumors of the adrenal cortex is surgical. Unfortunately, these tumors are rarely completely resectable at the time of the initial operation. In the nonresectable tumors, two types of therapeutic approaches have been used: the first is interference with steroid hormone synthesis for relief of the symptoms of Cushing's syndrome; the second is the use of cytotoxic chemotherapeutic agents.

Tryparanol and metapyrone, inhibitors of steroid hormone synthesis, have been tried without much success.[23, 24] At the present time, the therapeutic agent of choice in nonresectable adrenocortical carcinoma is o,p'-DDD, a compound related to the insecticide DDT. Its precise mechanism of action is uncertain but may be related to its lipid solubility.

The major toxic side effects of o,p'-DDD are gastrointestinal, neurologic, and dermatologic. This agent produces nausea and vomiting in a majority of patients, whether it is given orally or intravenously. Neurologic complications include drowsiness, depression, vertigo, and tremor. Skin rashes are seen in roughly one-third of patients.

The toxicity of o,p'-DDD generally imposes a limitation on the amount of drug that can be given. It is given in divided oral doses totaling 8 to 10 gm. per day. Smaller doses are given initially with gradual increments depending on the patient's tolerance of the drug. In responsive tumors, the drug may produce adrenal insufficiency, and dexamethasone should be used.

The clinical picture and the level of urinary adrenal hormones are guides to the effectiveness of o,p'-DDD. In 7 of 18 patients treated by Bergenstal et al.[25] at the National Cancer Institute, a fall in urinary adrenal hormone excretion was attended by clinical improvement. In an equal number of patients, the hormone excretion fell but there was no obvious clinical benefit. Remission may persist for periods of weeks to years. If the remission is achieved with o,p'-DDD, it is probably best to attempt to maintain it with reduced doses of the drug (2 to 4 mg. per day).

One interesting patient reported by Molnar et al.[26] was treated at the Mayo Clinic by multiple surgical procedures to remove isolated metastatic lesions, and then by prolonged therapy with o,p'-DDD. The patient had no detectable disease after 3½ years.

HORMONE-PRODUCING NONENDOCRINE TUMORS

A number of tumors not ordinarily thought to be endocrinologically active may on occasion produce a variety of hormones.[27, 28] The impressive variety of hormones they produce includes antidiuretic hormone,[29] ACTH,[30] gonadotropins,[31, 32] insulin-like activity,[33] growth hormone,[34] thyrocalcitonin,[35] erythropoietin,[36] and renin.[37] In addition, certain large tumors are associated with hypoglycemia without an elevated serum insulin level or insulin-like activity.[38] By far the most common "nonendocrine tumor" with endocrine activity has been bronchogenic carcinoma,[27, 29, 32] although renal cell carcinoma not infrequently has associated manifestations best explained on a humoral basis.[39]

The therapeutic approach to such endocrinologically active tumors must encompass both an attack on the malignant disease and control of the manifestations of excess hormone production. Since these hormonally active tumors are relatively rare and each demands a separate approach, the interested reader should consult the original literature cited.

REFERENCES

1. Pheochromocytoma: Current concepts of diagnosis and treatment. Clinical Staff Conference. Ann. Intern. Med., 65:1302–1326, 1966.
2. Melmon, K. L.: Catecholamines and the adrenal medulla. In Williams, R. H. (Editor): Textbook of Endocrinology. Ed. 4. Philadelphia, W. B. Saunders Company, 1968, p. 379.
3. Phaeochromocytoma and thyroid cancer. [Lead article.] Brit. Med. J., 2:549, 1965.
4. Engleman, K., and Sjoerdsma, A.: Chronic medical therapy for pheochromocytoma. A report of four cases. Ann. Intern. Med., 61:229–241, 1964.
5. Roy, S. B., Bhatia, M. L., and Mathur, V. S.: Guanethidine and phaeochromocytoma. Brit. Med. J., 1:729–730, 1963.
6. Melmon, K. L.: The endocrinologic manifestations of the carcinoid tumor. In Williams, R. H. (Editor): Textbook of Endocrinology. Ed. 4. Philadelphia, W. B. Saunders Company, 1968, p. 1161.
7. Sjoerdsma, A., and Melmon, K. L.: The carcinoid spectrum. Gastroenterology, 47:104, 1964.
8. Mengel, C. E.: Therapy of the malignant carcinoid syndrome. Ann. Intern. Med., 62:587–602, 1965.
9. MacDonald, R. A.: A study of 356 carcinoids of the gastrointestinal tract. Amer. J. Med., 21:867–878, 1956.
10. Melmon, K. L., Sjoerdsma, A., and Mason, D. T.: Distinctive clinical and therapeutic aspects of the syndrome associated with bronchial carcinoid tumors. Amer. J. Med., 39:568–581, 1965.
11. Oates, J. A., and Sjoerdsma, A.: A unique syndrome associated with secretion of 5-hydroxytryptophan by metastatic gastric carcinoids. Amer. J. Med., 32:333–342, 1962.
12. Humoral basis of carcinoid flush. [Lead article.] Lancet, 2:1013, 1966.
13. Wilson, H., Butterick, O. D., Jr.: Massive liver resection for control of severe vasomotor reactions secondary to malignant carcinoid. Ann. Surg., 149:648, 1959.
14. Stanford, W. R., David, J. E., Gunter, J. U., and Hobart, S. A., Jr.: Bronchial adenoma (carcinoid type) with solitary metastasis and associated functioning carcinoid syndrome. Southern Med. J., 51:449, 1958.
15. Vaeth, J. M., Rousseau, R. E., and Purcell, T. R.: Radiation response of carcinoid of the rectum. A case report. Amer. J. Roentgenol., 88:967–970, 1962.
16. Ellis, F. W.: Carcinoid of the rectum: Report of a case of thirteen years' survival; Treated with intra-arterial nitrogen mustard. Cancer, 10:138–142, 1957.
17. Moertel, C. G., and Reitemeier, R. J.: Experience with 5-fluorouracil in the palliative management of advanced carcinoma of the gastrointestinal tract. Proc. Mayo Clin., 37:520–529, 1962.
18. Reed, M. L., et al.: Treatment of disseminated carcinoid tumors including hepatic-artery catheterization. New Eng. J. Med., 269:1005–1010, 1963.
19. Melmon, K. L., Sjoerdsma, A., Oates, J. A., and Laster, L.: Treatment of malabsorption and diarrhea of the carcinoid syndrome with methysergide. Gastroenterology, 48:18, 1965.
20. Engelman, K., Lovenber, W., and Sjoerdsma, A.: Inhibition of serotonin synthesis by para-chlorophenylalanine in patients with the carcinoid syndrome. New Eng. J. Med., 277:1103–1108, 1967.

21. Melmon, K. L., and Cline, M. J.: Kinins (editorial). Amer. J. Med., *43*:153–160, 1967.
22. Lipsett, M. B., Hertz, R., and Ross, G. T.: Clinical and pathophysiologic aspects of adrenocortical carcinoma. Amer. J. Med., *35*:374–383, 1963.
23. Melby, J. C., St. Cyr, M., and Dale, S. L.: Reduction of adrenal-steroid production by an inhibitor of cholesterol biosynthesis. New Eng. J. Med., *264*:583–587, 1961.
24. Fukushima, D. K., Gallagher, T. F., Greenberg, W., and Pearson, O. H.: Studies with an adrenal inhibitor in adrenal carcinoma. J. Clin. Endocrinology, *20*:1234–1245, 1960.
25. Bergenstal, D. M., Hertz, R., Lipsett, M. B., and Moy, R. H.: Chemotherapy of adrenocortical cancer with o,p'-DDD. Ann. Intern. Med., *53*:672–682, 1960.
26. Molnar, G. D., Mattox, V. R., and Bahn, R. C.: Clinical and therapeutic observations in adrenal cancer: A report on 7 patients treated with o,p'-DDD. Cancer, *16*:259–268, 1963.
27. Bower, B. F., and Gordan, G. S.: Hormonal effects of nonendocrine tumors. Ann. Rev. Med., *16*:83–118, 1965.
28. Knowles, J. H., and Smith, L. H., Jr.: Extrapulmonary manifestations of bronchogenic carcinoma. New Eng. J. Med., *262*:505–510, 1960.
29. Bartter, F. C., and Schwartz, W. B.: The syndrome of inappropriate secretion of antidiuretic hormone. Amer. J. Med., *42*:790–806, 1967.
30. O'Riordan, J. L., Blanshard, G. P., Moxham, A., and Nabarro, J. D. N.: Corticotrophin-secreting carcinomas. Quart. J. Med., *35*:137–147, 1966.
31. Fusco, F. D., and Rosen, S. W.: Gonadotropin-producing anaplastic large-cell carcinomas of the lung. New Eng. J. Med., *275*:507, 1966.
32. Faiman, C., Colwell, J. A., Ryan, R. J., Hershman, J. M., and Shields, T. W.: Gonadotropin secretion from a bronchogenic carcinoma. New Eng. J. Med., *277*:1395–1399, 1967.
33. Unger, R. H.: The riddle of tumor hypoglycemia (editorial). Amer. J. Med., *40*:325–330, 1966.
34. Steiner, H., Dahlbäck, O., and Waldenström, J.: Ectopic growth-hormone production and osteoarthropathy in carcinoma of the bronchus. Lancet, *1*:783, 1968.
35. Meyer, J. S., and Abdel-Bari, W.: Granules and thyrocalcitonin-like activity in medullary carcinoma of the thyroid gland. New Eng. J. Med., *278*:523, 1968.
36. Waldmann, T. A., Rosse, W. F., and Swarm, R. L.: The erythropoiesis-stimulating factors produced by tumors. Ann. New York Acad. Sci., *149*:509, 1968.
37. Robertson, P. W., et al.: Hypertension due to a renin-secreting renal tumour. Amer. J. Med., *43*:963–976, 1967.
38. Nissan, S., Bar-Maor, A., and Shafrir, E.: Hypoglycemia associated with extrapancreatic tumors. New Eng. J. Med., *278*:177–183, 1968.
39. Extrarenal manifestations of hypernephroma. Medical Staff Conference, California Med., *109*:35–40, 1968.

Additional Recent Bibliography Not Cited in Text

40. Huvos, A. G., Hajdu, S. I., Brasfield, R. D., and Foote, F. W., Jr.: Adrenal cortical carcinoma. Clinicopathologic study of 34 cases. Cancer, *25*:354–361, 1970.
41. Colin-Jones, D. G., Gibbs, D. D., Copping, R. M. L., and Sharr, M. M.: Malignant Zollinger-Ellison syndrome with gastrin-containing skin metastases. Lancet, *1*:492–494, 1969.
42. McFadzean, A. J. S., and Yeung, R. T. T.: Further observations on hypoglycaemia in hepatocellular carcinoma. Amer. J. Med., *47*:220–235, 1969.

CHAPTER 9

MALIGNANT TUMORS OF CHILDHOOD (SOLID TUMORS)

Malignancy is rare in childhood compared to malignancy in adults. Notwithstanding, cancer is a leading cause of death due to disease in children over one year of age[1] and it is second only to death due to accidents. The incidence of pediatric cancer peaks twice: during the first six years of life and during adolescence.

Acute leukemia accounts for one-third to one-half of all malignant tumors of childhood. Brain tumors are next in frequency. Wilms' tumor, neuroblastoma, soft tissue sarcomas, and Ewing's sarcoma each account for 5 to 10 per cent of childhood malignancies.[1] This chapter is concerned with the solid tumors of childhood. Acute lymphoblastic leukemia in children is considered in Chapter 10.

Certain differences in the patterns of malignant disease in children and adults are of interest. A large proportion of the malignancies of childhood are of hematopoietic origin, whereas the commonest adult tumors are of epithelial origin. The characteristics of the tumor that are considered predictive of a benign or malignant course in adults are often not prognostic signs in childhood neoplasms. For example, in adults encapsulation of a malignant tumor is often considered to be a good prognostic sign; in children neuroblastoma and Wilms' tumor may be wholly encapsulated and be exceedingly malignant. Mitotic figures and invasion of surrounding structures frequently may be seen in relatively benign childhood tumors such as hemangiomas, but they are usually associated with malignant disease in adults. It is also apparent that the response to chemotherapy may be related to age. For example, acute leukemia is more responsive to chemotherapy in childhood than in adult life. Cures of Wilms' tumor and neuroblastoma predominate in children under one year of age.

WILMS' TUMOR

Good reviews of the natural history and pathologic characteristics of Wilms' tumor (embryonal sarcoma of kidney) are available.[2, 3] Wilms' tumor is one of the common solid tumors of childhood. It may be present at birth and usually involves a single kidney, although both kidneys are involved in 1 to 5 per cent of the patients. The diagnosis is usually made before the age of 5. At the time of diagnosis, 10 to 20 per cent of patients have evidence of distant metastasis and often multiple metastases. The most common sites of metastases are the lungs; less common sites are the brain, liver, and bone. The tumor is encapsulated; it usually has both sarcomatous and carcinomatous elements, and may have striated muscle and smooth muscle as well. If the tumor breaks through its capsule, it usually invades the renal veins, renal pelvis, and ureters. If the capsule is broken at the time of surgery, local recurrence is common.

An important consideration in the treatment of this neoplasm is that *if the child is apparently free of metastases two years after treatment, cure is virtually certain.*[4] This means that careful follow-up examination, including chest roentgenograms and renal function studies, is mandatory. The initial evaluation includes chest roentgenograms, intravenous pyelogram, and inferior vena cavagram.

The sequential therapeutic approach to the patient with unilateral Wilms' tumor is outlined in Figure 9–1. A relatively recent innovation in the primary therapy of Wilms' tumor is the combination of surgery, radiation therapy, and chemotherapy; a much higher rate of

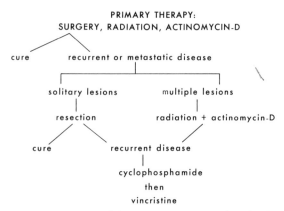

Figure 9–1   Sequence of therapy in patients with Wilms' tumor.

cure has been obtained than that previously obtained by means of traditional treatment with surgery or radiation therapy alone.[4, 5] Farber[4] found that this multidisciplinary combination therapy apparently cured more than 80 per cent of those with disseminated disease.

It cannot be emphasized too strongly that *a vigorous attack with the combined weapons of surgery, radiation therapy, and chemotherapy is indicated even when the disease appears to be hopelessly disseminated.* Cures may be achieved even in the presence of widespread metastases (see illustrative case history). Even involvement of both kidneys by the malignancy does not preclude therapy with the objective of cure, provided a suitable renal transplant donor is available.

The surgical management of Wilms' tumor has been outlined by Gross.[6] After surgery, the tumor bed and involved lungs are treated with x-ray therapy at a dose below the level that will induce radiation pneumonitis or nephritis. Farber[4] has recently undertaken a program in which the radiation therapy is omitted whenever possible in infants under one year of age, in order to avoid subsequent skeletal abnormalities. The long-term results of such a program are still unknown, and most institutions consider x-irradiation as part of "standard" therapy.

The primary chemotherapy given at the time of surgery is a course of actinomycin-D, 15 μg. per kg. on each of 5 successive days (total dosage, 75 μg. per kg. for a single course). Somewhat smaller doses are used in small infants. Recently a controlled cooperative study has shown that the rate of recurrence is considerably lower in patients given maintenance therapy with actinomycin-D intermittently (every 3 months for 15 months) than in patients receiving a single course of the drug.[7] On such a maintenance program, toxicity has been minimal; nausea and vomiting are the chief problems. The results of the intermittent therapy program are sufficiently impressive to recommend it as the best approach at present.

At the time of initial treatment the tumor may be so large as to make surgery hazardous. In such cases, the tumor may be reduced by preoperative irradiation or by administering vincristine. Single doses of vincristine of 0.05 mg. per kg. or higher have been used with success.[8, 9]

In patients with recurrent or metastatic disease after primary treatment, radiation therapy and actinomycin-D should still be considered the best therapeutic modalities, offering the possibility of cure. When they have been used without response, or if toxicity intervenes, vincristine should be considered, and subsequently cyclophosphamide. Approximately one-third of patients with disseminated disease can be expected to show a partial response to a regimen of cyclophosphamide, 5 mg. per kg. intravenously for 10 days, followed by daily oral doses of 2.5 to 5 mg. per kg.[10]

An experimental drug, tryptophan mustard, has also been reported to have produced a partial response in a patient with Wilms' tumor.[11]

NEUROBLASTOMA

The natural history and results of treatment of neuroblastoma have been reviewed recently.[12] Occasionally confusion arises in the diagnosis of neuroblastoma. The principal malignancies that may resemble neuroblastoma include Ewing's sarcoma, poorly differentiated sarcomas, and reticulum cell sarcoma. The peak incidence of this disease occurs within the first three years of life, and in more than 50 per cent of cases the diagnosis is made before the age of 2. In more than half the patients, metastases are evident at the time of diagnosis. The primary neoplasm may be anywhere between the head and the pelvis, but over half are in the adrenal gland and three fourths in the retroperitoneal space. About 10 per cent are found in the mediastinum.

A thorough evaluation of the patient with this tumor includes an intravenous pyelogram, a chest roentgenogram, an inferior vena cavagram, and bone marrow aspiration. Marrow aspirate contains tumor cells in about 40 per cent of patients. Some of these tumors (of sympathetic nervous system origin) synthesize catecholamines, and catecholamine metabolites such as vanylmandelic acid may appear in the urine.

The primary therapy for neuroblastoma is surgical extirpation. Often radiation therapy is used preoperatively to reduce a tumor to a surgically manageable size. Some investigators also use irradiation postoperatively.[12]

It seems clear that aggressive attempts to remove the primary tumor are indicated. When excision is not possible at an initial operation, radiation therapy may alter the situation so that the tumor may be successfully removed at a second operation. Initial x-irradiation may also allow preservation of viscera adjacent to the tumor at the time of surgery.

The major prognostic factors are the degree of differentiation of the tumor and the completeness of surgical removal.[12] About 50 per cent of the tumors show no evidence of differentiation beyond the presence of rosettes. The lack of differentiation carries a grave prognosis, but the presence of a high degree of differentiation does not guarantee the success of therapy. Differentiated tumors are more common in younger children. In a series of patients treated by surgery and local radiation therapy without concomitant chemotherapy, Gross et al.[13] achieved a cure rate of 88 per cent in patients with completely resectable tumor. Palliative excision or biopsy alone

TABLE 9–1 *Chemotherapy of Disseminated Neuroblastoma*

DRUG	DOSE SCHEDULE	CHIEF MANIFESTATIONS OF TOXICITY
Cyclophosphamide	5 mg./kg./day x 10 I.V.; then 2.5 mg./kg./day orally	Bone marrow depression, hemorrhagic cystitis
Vincristine	2.5 mg./sq. M./week I.V.	Neuropathy, severe constipation

resulted in a cure rate of 64 per cent and 10 per cent, respectively. This high cure rate has generally not been matched in other series.

What are the criteria of cure in neuroblastoma? *No patient living and apparently free of metastases 5 years after treatment has died of this disease.* Evaluation of the effectiveness of therapy must take account of the occasional observations of spontaneous regression of metastases after local treatment of the primary tumor.[14]

Treatment of Disseminated Neuroblastoma

In the treatment of disseminated neuroblastoma, cyclophosphamide is the treatment of choice and produces a beneficial effect in roughly 80 per cent of patients (Table 9-1).[15] Daily oral therapy is superior to intermittent high-dose treatment. The suggested cyclophosphamide schedule is: 5 mg. per kg. per day intravenously for 10 days, then a daily oral maintenance dosage of 2.5 mg. per kg. The dose must be reduced if neutropenia occurs; the white blood cell count should not be permitted to fall below 3000 per cu. mm. The usual cyclophosphamide-associated toxic side effects, including bone marrow depression, gastrointestinal intolerance, alopecia, and hemorrhagic cystitis, may be encountered. These complications are usually avoidable or of minor intensity when therapy is carefully controlled.

An alternative to cyclophosphamide therapy is vincristine in weekly doses of 2.5 mg. per sq. M.[16] or 0.05 to 0.075 mg. per kg.[17] A response rate of 30 to 50 per cent may be anticipated. Combined therapy with vincristine and cyclophosphamide has been tried, but it is too early to evaluate the results of this combination.

Vitamin B_{12} has been used in treating neuroblastoma, but a survey of this experience does not support the use of this agent in therapy.[18] Its use merely delays definitive treatment.

EWING'S SARCOMA

Ewing's sarcoma is a malignant tumor of bone usually occurring during the first two decades of life and showing a predilection for males. Reviews of series of cases of Ewing's sarcoma are available.[19, 20] The mortality is high; in one extensive series of cases, 85 per cent of patients were dead within 2 years after diagnosis.[21] However, other recent reports are somewhat more optimistic.[22] The pattern of metastases is to lung, bone, and lymph nodes.

Most authorities agree that radiation therapy is the chief modality of primary treatment of this disease.[22, 23] Radical radiation therapy combined with total-body irradiation has been reported.[23] A few centers still use surgery when the primary tumor occurs in a resectable area.

The advantage of using chemotherapy in association with radiation therapy as the primary treatment of this neoplasm is not definitely established; however, some interesting preliminary reports exist. Vincristine and cyclophosphamide in combination with radiation therapy have been used in a small series of patients, with impressive results.[24, 25]

In the treatment of disseminated disease, cyclophosphamide (15 mg. per kg. intravenously once weekly) has received the most extensive trial and has produced responses in roughly 65 per cent of a small series of patients.[26] Similar results have been reported when smaller doses have been used.[27] The drug may also be given intrapleurally in the treatment of recurrent effusions.

Melphalan and vincristine have produced results distinctly inferior to those of cyclophosphamide in small series of patients.[17, 26] Actinomycin-D may be useful in occasional patients who are refractory to cyclophosphamide.[28]

It is worth stressing that an aggressive approach is indicated even in the presence of demonstrable metastases. The combination of radiation therapy and chemotherapy, and sometimes judicious surgery, may produce a prolonged remission and even an occasional cure.

SOFT TISSUE SARCOMAS

Soft tissue sarcomas account for approximately 10 per cent of the malignant tumors of childhood.[29] They occur throughout all the years of childhood. The most common sites are the head, neck, and pelvis. They may be associated with a high incidence of congenital anomalies.[30] In a series of 135 cases, rhabdomyosarcomas accounted for 56 per cent and sarcoma of undetermined histogenesis for 20 per cent of all soft tissue sarcomas in the pediatric age range.[31]

Rhabdomyosarcomas are generally classified into four types: pleomorphic, alveolar, embryonal, and botryoid.[32] The last three types are more common in children than in adults and are thought to be pathologic variants of the same tumor.[33] Pleomorphic rhabdomyo-sarcoma, in contrast, is a disease of late adult life.[34]

Surgery is the primary therapeutic modality in the soft tissue sarcomas of childhood, usually combined with radiation therapy. These tumors are often radiosensitive in childhood, whereas they are usually radioresistant in adults. The well-differentiated sarcomas of childhood, including fibrosarcoma, liposarcoma, and certain rhabdo-myosarcomas, are usually radioresistant. Nelson[33] has shown that embryonal rhabdomyosarcoma is often moderately radiosensitive and can be locally controlled for significant periods of time by radiation therapy.

The optimal chemotherapeutic schedule for soft tissue sarcomas in childhood has not been established. Mention is made in the literature of actinomycin-D and vincristine therapy, but the data are insufficient for evaluation.[16] Two recent reports describe dramatic results in the treatment of rhabdomyosarcoma with response rates of 80 to 100 per cent. Combination chemotherapy with vincristine, actinomycin-D, and cyclophosphamide produced complete or partial response in each of 7 patients, with a median duration of response of 4.5 months (range 1.5 to 18 months).[35] Another investigator, describing his experience with weekly high-dose cyclophosphamide (30 mg. per kg. intravenously or orally), reported good or partial responses in 11 of 14 patients, with a median duration of response of 2.5 months (range, 1 to 8.5 months).[10] These reports, although preliminary, are encouraging.

ILLUSTRATIVE CASE HISTORY: DISSEMINATED WILMS' TUMOR

The patient's clinical course is summarized in Figure 9-2.

A boy aged 3 years and 9 months entered a community hospital in *May 1967* because of hematuria and a palpable abdominal mass. A malignancy was suspected. At surgery, a well-encapsulated Wilms' tumor (3 by 4 cm.) was found and a left nephrectomy was performed. No evidence of metastatic disease was observed at the time of this surgery. Postoperatively the child was given a 5-day course of actinomycin-D (total dose, 60 μg. per kg.). X-ray therapy of the tumor bed was begun but was soon discontinued because of the patient's intolerance of the therapy.

In *August 1967*, pulmonary metastases were found, and the patient was treated with 1500 rads to both lung fields over a 6-week period and 3 more courses of actinomycin-D over a 3-month period. After this therapy, the patient felt well for about 2 months. However, in *February 1968*, he was referred to the University of California Hospitals, San Francisco, with symptoms of anorexia and an enlarging abdomen. A right upper quadrant mass was felt, and abnormal liver function was detected. A partial hepatectomy was performed, and a mass in the right lobe of the liver was partially ex-

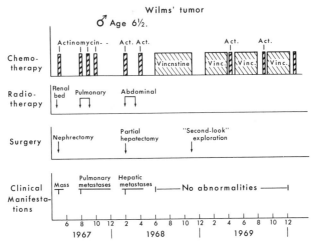

Figure 9–2 Summary of the therapy and clinical course of a patient with disseminated Wilms' tumor. See case history.

cised. Postoperative radiation therapy was given to a large abdominal field, including the liver, over a period of 6 weeks. Actinomycin-D was given again in two 5-day courses, each totaling 75 μg. per kg.

Despite this therapy, abnormalities of liver function persisted and the child's clinical course deteriorated. Therefore, in *June* 1968, treatment with vincristine, 1 mg. per week, was begun and continued for 3 months; the drug dose was then reduced to 1 mg. every other week. The patient tolerated this therapy well, although he developed alopecia, complained of anorexia, and had poor weight gain. During this time, no other evidence of metastatic disease was found by chest roentgenograms or intravenous pyelogram.

In *November 1968*, a "second look" laparotomy was performed to explore the site of the original tumor and evaluate the completeness of eradication of the hepatic metastasis. No recurrent malignant disease was found in the left renal fossa, and only scar tissue and focal hepatocellular necrosis were found in a large biopsy specimen of the liver.

After this operation, a program of cyclic chemotherapy was begun. The program consisted of vincristine, 1 mg. every other week for 3 months, followed by 2 weeks without therapy, and then a 5-day course of actinomycin-D totaling 75 μg. per kg. Thereafter, the cycle was repeated. At the present time, the patient has been on this program for 18 months, and is still on it. The program is to be continued until the patient has been free of tumor for 2 years. At present, he is free of any disease as judged by physical examination, roentgenologic studies (including roentgenograms, bone surveys, and intravenous pyelogram), and liver function tests. Despite administration of large amounts of vincristine, the patient has not developed evidence of neuropathy. The results of blood studies have been within normal limits.

In the past 15 months, the boy (now almost 7 years of age) has gained 4 kg. in weight and 12 cm. in height. He is active and is apparently healthy.

COMMENT: This child with Wilms' tumor of the left kidney was treated initially with surgery, actinomycin-D, and limited radiation therapy. When pulmonary metastatic lesions appeared, they were treated with radiation and chemotherapy. Despite subsequent courses of actinomycin-D, hepatic metastases developed. This tumor was partially excised and also irradiated, and the patient was placed on a program of alternating vincristine and actinomycin-D. No evidence of malignant disease has been found since *June 1968*. This case exemplifies the vigorous attack by surgery, radiation therapy, and chemotherapy indicated in treating Wilms' tumor, even when it is disseminated.

REFERENCES

1. Murphy, M. L.: Curability of cancer in children. Cancer, 22:779–784, 1968.
2. Ariel, J. M., and Pack, G. T.: Cancer and Allied Diseases of Infancy and Childhood. Boston, Little, Brown and Company, 1960.
3. Willis, R. A.: The Pathology of the Tumours of Children. Springfield, Illinois, Charles C Thomas, 1962.
4. Farber, S.: Chemotherapy in the treatment of leukemia and Wilms' tumor. J.A.M.A., 198:154, 1966.
5. Fernbach, D. J., and Martyn, D. T.: Role of dactinomycin in the improved survival of children with Wilms' tumor. J.A.M.A., 195:1005–1009, 1966.
6. Gross, R. E.: The Surgery of Infancy and Childhood. Philadelphia, W. B. Saunders Company, 1957, p. 597.
7. Wolff, J. A., Krivit, W., Newton, W. A., Jr., and D'Angio, G. J.: Single versus multiple dose dactinomycin therapy of Wilms's tumor. New Eng. J. Med., 279:290, 1968.
8. Sullivan, M. P., Sutow, W. W., Cangir, A., and Taylor, G.: Vincristine sulfate in management of Wilms' tumor. J.A.M.A., 202:381–384, 1967.
9. Sullivan, M. P.: Vincristine (NSC-67574) therapy for Wilms' tumor. Cancer Chemother. Rep., 52:481–484, 1968.
10. Sutow, W. W.: Cyclophosphamide (NSC-26271) in Wilms' tumor and rhabdomyosarcoma. Cancer Chemother. Rep., 51:407–409, 1967.
11. Kung, F., et al.: Tryptophan mustard (NSC-62403) in the treatment of acute leukemia and malignant solid tumors in children. Cancer Chemother. Rep., 52:445-450, 1968.
12. Fortner, J., Nicastri, A., and Murphy, M. L.: Neuroblastoma: Natural history and results of treating 133 cases. Ann. Surg., 167:132–142, 1968.
13. Gross, R. E., Farber, S., and Martin, L. W.: Neuroblastoma sympatheticum. A study and report of 217 cases. Pediatrics, 23:1179, 1959.
14. Kontras, S. B.: Urinary excretion of 3-methoxy-4-hydroxymandelic acid in children with neuroblastoma. Cancer, 15:978–986, 1962.
15. Thurman, W. G., and Donaldson, M. H.: Cyclophosphamide (NSC-26271) therapy for children with neuroblastoma. Cancer Chemother. Rep., 51:399–401, 1967.
16. Selawry, O. S., Holland, J. F., and Wolman, I. J.: Effect of vincristine (NSC-67574) on malignant solid tumors in children. Cancer Chemother. Rep., 52:497–500, 1968.
17. Sutow, W. W.: Vincristine (NSC-67574) therapy for malignant solid tumors in children (except Wilms' tumor). Cancer Chemother. Rep., 52:485–487, 1968.
18. Sawitsky, A., and Desposito, F.: A survey of American experience with vitamin B_{12} therapy of neuroblastoma. J. Pediat., 67:99–103, 1965.
19. Bhansali, S. K., and Desai, P. B.: Ewing's sarcoma. Observations on 107 cases. J. Bone Joint Surg., 45(A):541, 1963.
20. Dahlin, D. C., Coventry, M. D., and Scanlon, P. W.: Ewing's sarcoma—a critical analysis of 165 cases. J. Bone Joint Surg., 43(A):185, 1961.

21. Falk, S., and Alpert, M.: Five year survival of patients with Ewing's sarcoma. Surg. Gynec. Obst., 124:319–324, 1967.
22. Phillips, R. F., and Higinbotham, N. L.: The curability of Ewing's endothelioma of bone in children. J. Pediat., 70:391–397, 1967.
23. Millburn, L. F., O'Grady, L., and Hendrickson, F. R.: Radical radiation therapy and total body irradiation in the treatment of Ewing's sarcoma. Cancer, 22:919–925, 1968.
24. Hustu, H. O., Holton, C., James, D., Jr., and Pinkel, D.: Treatment of Ewing's sarcoma with concurrent radiotherapy and chemotherapy. J. Pediat., 73:249–251, 1968.
25. Johnson, R., and Humphreys, S. R.: Past failures and future possibilities in Ewing's sarcoma. Experimental and preliminary clinical results. Cancer, 23:161–166, 1969.
26. Samuels, M. L., and Howe, C. D.: Cyclophosphamide in the management of Ewing's sarcoma. Cancer, 20:961–966, 1967.
27. Haggard, M. E.: Cyclophosphamide (NSC-26271) in the treatment of children with malignant neoplasms. Cancer Chemother. Rep., 51:403–405, 1967.
28. Evans, A. E.: Chemotherapy of solid tumors in children. In Brodsky, I., Kahn, S. B., Moyer, J. H. (Editors): Cancer Chemotherapy. New York, Grune & Stratton, Inc., 1967, p. 133.
29. Lawrence, E. A., and Donlan, E. J.: Neoplastic diseases in infants and children. Cancer Res., 12:900, 1952.
30. Sloane, J. A., and Hubbell, M. M.: Soft tissue sarcomas in children associated with congenital anomalies. Cancer, 23:175–182, 1969.
31. Soule, E. H., Mahour, G. H., Mills, S. D., and Lynn, H. B.: Soft-tissue sarcomas of infants and children: A clinicopathologic study of 135 cases. Proc. Mayo Clin., 43:313–326, 1968.
32. Horn, R. C., Jr., and Enterline, H. T.: Rhabdomyosarcoma: A clinicopathological study and classification of 39 cases. Cancer, 11:181, 1953.
33. Nelson, A. J., III: Embryonal rhabdomyosarcoma. Cancer, 22:64–68, 1968.
34. Keyhani, A., and Booher, R. J.: Pleomorphic rhabdomyosarcoma. Cancer, 22:956–967, 1968.
35. Pratt, C. B., James, D. H., Jr., Holton, C. P., and Pinkel, D.: Combination therapy including vincristine (NSC-67574) for malignant solid tumors in children. Cancer Chemother. Rep., 52:489–495, 1968.

Recent Additional Bibliography Not Cited in Text

36. Fraumeni, J. F., and Miller, R. W.: Cancer deaths in the newborn. Amer. J. Dis. Child., 117:186–189, 1969.
37. Tefft, M.: Radioisotopes in malignancies in children. J.A.M.A., 207:1853–1858, 1969.
38. Vietti, T. J., Sullivan, M. P., Haggard, M. E., Holcomb, T. M., and Berry, D. H.: Vincristine sulfate and radiation therapy in metastatic Wilms' tumor. Cancer, 25:12–20, 1970.

CHAPTER 10

ACUTE LEUKEMIA

In no area of cancer chemotherapy has the research activity been as intense and the results as dramatic and encouraging as in acute leukemia. In recent years there has been consistent application of principles derived from experimental models and animal research to the problems of the clinic.[1, 2] Use of new drugs, improved dosage schedules, combination therapy, and intensive supportive therapy have been reflected in the prolongation of survival in patients with acute lymphocytic leukemia.[3, 4] This effect is not as clearly demonstrable in life-table analyses of patients with acute myelocytic leukemia, but such analyses do not tell the whole story of the recent advances in the control of this form of acute leukemia.

TYPES OF ACUTE LEUKEMIA

At the outset, it is important to distinguish and catalogue the various types of acute leukemia morphologically, by natural history, and by response to treatment. In Table 10-1, I have attempted a classification of the major morphologic types and variants of acute leukemia. Not all authorities agree to any one uniform classification of the acute leukemias. Some do not acknowledge the existence of forms that defy precise morphologic classification into either the lymphocytic or granulocytic series (i.e., undifferentiated acute leukemia). Others are impressed by monocytic leukemia as a distinct disease entity.

In practical terms, however, there is a group of patients with acute leukemia whose disease is difficult to classify morphologically, accounting for 10 to 15 per cent of all patients with acute leukemia. They are best considered as either acute undifferentiated leukemia of childhood, equivalent to acute lymphocytic leukemia, or as acute

TABLE 10-1 *Classification of Acute Leukemia*

MAJOR MORPHOLOGIC TYPE AND VARIANTS	AGE (MAJORITY OF PATIENTS)	MEDIAN SURVIVAL	APPROXIMATE RATE OF FIRST REMISSION
Acute lymphocytic leukemia	Children and young adults	14 to >24 months, depending on treatment center	90%
Undifferentiated leukemia of childhood "Stem cell" leukemia of childhood			
Acute myelocytic leukemia Promyelocytic leukemia Myelomonocytic leukemia Undifferentiated acute leukemia of adults Monocytic leukemia	Chiefly adults	Generally <8 months	10–35%

leukemia of adults, equivalent to acute myelocytic leukemia. On the basis of clinical manifestations or responsiveness to treatment, there is no need to subdivide morphologic variants of acute myelocytic leukemia, myelomonocytic leukemia, or monocytic leukemia. Therefore, for practical purposes, all of these can be considered as acute myelocytic leukemia. The morphologic criteria for distinguishing these types of cells are available in the literature.[5, 6]

MANIFESTATIONS

The major manifestations of acute leukemia, acute lymphocytic leukemia, or acute myelocytic leukemia result from proliferation of the neoplastic cells and concomitant injury to normal tissues. These are:

1. Derangements due to loss of normal bone marrow elements: anemia (red cell precursors); granulocytopenia, infection (granulocyte precursors); thrombocytopenia, bleeding (platelet precursors).
2. Leukemic infiltration, malfunctioning of specific organs: liver, central nervous system, bone, lung.
3. Metabolic abnormalities: hyperuricemia, hypercalcemia, fever.

Loss of normal bone marrow elements is critical to the clinical manifestations of leukemia and is brought about either by physical crowding or, more likely, by competition with the malignant cells for biochemical substrates.

Anemia results from both inadequate erythropoiesis and a shortened red cell lifespan. Morphologic abnormalities of the red cells in the peripheral blood are common.

Also common are granulocytopenia (with increased susceptibility to infection) and thrombocytopenia (with a consequent bleeding tendency). As a rule of thumb, propensity to infection increases as the absolute neutrophil count falls below 600 per cu. mm. This figure may be used as a guide to determine whether isolation procedures are necessary for the patient. Similarly, bleeding problems can be anticipated when the platelet count falls below 50,000 per cu. mm.

Almost every organ system shows microscopic evidence of leukemic infiltration. Clinically obvious organ malfunction is unusual, however, except in the case of the liver, central nervous system, lung, and bone. Bone pain is frequent, and sternal tenderness is often a good guide to leukemia in relapse. Rarely osteolysis is associated with hypercalcemia.

The hyperuricemia and increased urinary excretion of uric acid are easy to understand in view of the greatly increased nucleic acid turnover. Less easy to understand is the fever that often accompanies acute leukemia. In roughly one-half to two-thirds of the patients with fever, a microbial origin can be demonstrated by culture, serology, or responsiveness of the fever to antibiotic therapy. In the remaining patients no microbial cause can be demonstrated.

A point worth noting is that the clinical manifestations of acute leukemia are subtle or undetectable until the body burden of leukemic cells exceeds approximately 10^{10}. When the cell number reaches about 10^{12}, the disease picture is full blown.[3, 7]

OBJECTIVES OF THERAPY

What are the objectives of treatment in acute leukemia? Most physicians would agree that the objectives of treatment are an improvement in the feeling of well-being of the patient and a prolongation of life. In acute lymphocytic leukemia there is a good correlation among survival, sense of well-being, and the induction of the first hematologic remission. (In acute myelocytic leukemia this correlation is not as good.) Therefore, *in acute lymphocytic leukemia the chief objective of therapy is the induction of complete hematologic remission,* i.e., return of blood and bone marrow to normal status and disappearance of any evidence of compromised organ function.

In acute myelocytic leukemia the objectives of treatment are similar, but the physician often must be content with a partial remission, i.e., incomplete disappearance of leukemic cells and partial recovery of normal blood and marrow elements and organ function.

As chemotherapy has become more aggressive, another objective has been to reduce the body burden of leukemic cells to the lowest possible levels. These levels can be estimated only indirectly.[3, 5]

SUPPORTIVE THERAPY

Two types of therapy must be considered: specific chemotherapy and intensive supportive care. Bleeding and infection are the major clinical problems leading to death of the patient with acute leukemia. Supportive care, which has become increasingly important as part of total care, includes replacement of platelets, white blood cells, and red blood cells; the use of antibiotics; sterile precautions; and the use of xanthine oxidase inhibitors to control hyperuricemia.

It is obvious that if the physician could replace platelets and white blood cells with complete freedom, he could sustain patients with leukemia for a considerable length of time. It is already theoretically, and sometimes practically, possible to replace platelets. When platelets are given to the thrombocytopenic patient, they must be given soon enough and in adequate numbers: a minimum of 8 to 10 units for an adult, often at 48- to 72-hour intervals. One does not wait until the patient is bleeding actively before giving the platelets; by then it is generally too late. Therefore, the guideline is a platelet count of less than 30,000 per cu. mm. and peripheral manifestations of recent bleeding into skin or the buccal or nasal mucosa.

Infusion of white blood cells can be quite effective in patients with granulocytopenia and infections that are unresponsive to antibiotic therapy. This fact was first demonstrated by the studies at the National Cancer Institute, where leukocytes of patients with chronic myelocytic leukemia were given to children with acute leukemia who had infections (often *Pseudomonas*) that were unresponsive to antibiotic treatment. Not infrequently there was a dramatic clearing of these infections. Detailed studies demonstrated that the donor white cells persisted for reasonable periods, often for several months. Evidence of persistence was based on analysis of marrow karyotype for the Philadelphia chromosome. Unfortunately, leukocytes are not generally available for transfusion because of the difficulty and expense of obtaining them from normal subjects. It is likely, however, that they will become available in the not-too-distant future (see Chap. 15).

Supportive measures include the use of antibiotics, sterile precautions to prevent infection, and transfusion of red blood cells in the anemic patient. If an effective xanthine oxidase inhibitor with low toxicity (allopurinol) is used, hyperuricemia should not be a problem. Prevention of the renal complications of hyperuricemia is much easier than treatment of the established syndrome. Before beginning chemotherapy it is usually necessary to give large volumes of fluid orally or intravenously in order to induce a large output of urine. It is occasionally necessary to induce an alkaline urine (which increases the solubility of uric acid) by the administration of sodium bicarbonate.

Because the specific chemotherapeutic approaches to acute lymphocytic leukemia and acute myelocytic leukemia are so different, each is considered separately.

CHEMOTHERAPY OF ACUTE LYMPHOBLASTIC LEUKEMIA

Various kinds of agents have proved to be useful when used alone in inducing or maintaining remissions in acute lymphocytic leukemia (Table 10-2; refs. 9 to 21). They comprise two groups of agents, those in common use with well-established dosage schedules (standard) and those that are still experimental. Such a division is of necessity arbitrary in a field that is rapidly changing; however, the standard agents are widely available, whereas the experimental agents are presently restricted to approved clinical research centers.

Standard Agents

Certain drugs are effective in rapidly inducing a hematologic remission but not in maintaining a remission. Other agents induce remissions slowly or infrequently but are useful in maintenance therapy. This division into "inducers" and "maintainers" must also be considered arbitrary. As new dosage schedules are developed and

TABLE 10-2   Drugs Used in Treatment of Acute Lymphocytic Leukemia

DRUG	INDUCTION OR MAINTENANCE OF REMISSION	DOSAGE SCHEDULES	REMISSION INDUCTION RATE (%)	REFER-ENCE
Standard				
Corticosteroids	Induction	2–4 mg./kg./day p.o. (children); 60–120 mg./day (adults)	50–70	9
6-Mercaptopurine	Maintenance; sometimes induction	70–90 mg./sq. M./day p.o. (children); 2–2.5 mg./kg./day (adults)	30–40	8, 10
Methotrexate	Maintenance; also induction with intensive therapy	1. 3 mg./sq. M./day p.o. 2. 30 mg./sq. M. every 4 days	20	11–14
Vincristine	Induction	1–2 mg./sq. M./wk. I.V. (children); 0.025–0.05 mg./kg./wk. I.V. (adults)	50–80	15, 16
Cyclophosphamide	Induction; sometimes maintenance	100 mg./sq. M./day p.o.	15–20	17
Experimental				
Cytosine arabinoside	Induction	Under investigation	?	18
Daunomycin	Induction	Under investigation	? 10–30	19
BCNU°	Maintenance	Under investigation	?	20
L-asparaginase	Induction	Under investigation	? 50	21

° 1, 3-bis(β-chloroethyl)-1-nitrosourea.

drugs are used more effectively, the dividing line between the two categories of inducers and maintainers is becoming less distinct. For example, methotrexate, a "maintainer," may be a fairly effective inducing agent if administered intensively at high doses.

How does the physician decide which drug or which combination of potentially useful drugs to choose? My choice of conservative sequential chemotherapy of acute lymphocytic leukemia is summarized in Table 10-3. The best initial treatment is a combination of vincristine and prednisone for 4 to 6 weeks. With this regimen one can induce a remission well over 80 per cent of the time. Daily prednisone therapy is superior to treatment on alternate days.[9] Once remission has been induced, the steroid dose is reduced gradually and then administration is stopped and vincristine is discontinued. 6-Mercaptopurine is used as the first "maintenance" agent. The duration of maintained remission is somewhat longer with 6-mercaptopurine than with methotrexate. 6-Mercaptopurine used alone is as effective in maintaining a remission as a series of drugs given sequentially or cyclically.[10]

Therapy with 6-mercaptopurine is continued until relapse. After the first relapse of disease, the patient is usually treated again with prednisone or a combination of prednisone and vincristine. If a second remission is achieved, maintenance therapy is reinstituted, this time with methotrexate. If a second remission is not achieved with prednisone and vincristine, several alternatives are available: other standard agents may be considered, combination chemotherapy may be tried, or experimental drugs may be used if these are available (Table 10-3), e.g., cytosine arabinoside or daunomycin. These are also the alternatives to be considered after subsequent relapses following the second remission.

After the first relapse, the choice of agents is a matter of clinical

TABLE 10-3 *Sequential Chemotherapy of Acute Lymphocytic Leukemia*

1. Initial treatment	Prednisone plus vincristine to induce first remission; 6-Mercaptopurine to maintain remission.
2. Relapse	Prednisone or Prednisone plus vincristine to induce second remission; Methotrexate to maintain remission.
3. Relapse	Prednisone Vincristine, 6-Mercaptopurine, Cyclophosphamide, Cytosine arabinoside,° Daunomycin,° or Combinations of agents } to induce third and subsequent remissions

°Experimental.

judgment. When standard therapy has failed, the patient should be evaluated for treatment with experimental drug protocols. For this reason, some investigators have argued that all children with acute lymphocytic leukemia should be referred to special research centers for treatment.[3, 22]

Experimental Therapy

The major trends in experimental therapy of acute lymphocytic leukemia have been clearly summarized by Zubrod.[23] Briefly, these are the use of new agents, the use of established agents in new intensive dosage schedules (cf. ref. 24), and the vigorous use of combinations of cytotoxic agents.[25] Such methods rely heavily on experience derived from animal model systems[1, 2] and concepts of total numbers of leukemic cells.[23]

The combinations of several agents have produced results far superior to those achieved by single agents or a combination of two agents such as prednisone and vincristine. The interested reader can consult the original literature for the dosage schedules employed in combination therapy.[25-27] First, rapidly acting inducing agents (e.g., vincristine, prednisone, and daunomycin) are used for periods short of those that induce serious toxicity. Induction of remission is followed by the use of "consolidators," e.g., 6-mercaptopurine, methotrexate, cyclophosphamide, BCNU. "Reinduction" schedules are used periodically even when the child is in complete remission by all criteria. Such a schedule of "induction-consolidation-reinduction-consolidation" is part of the standard treatment protocol at several large treatment centers.

The place of new agents such as cytosine arabinoside and L-asparaginase in these combinations is still being evaluated. It is obvious that there are many possible combinations of the nine agents in Table 10-2 and of various dosage schedules. Novel approaches, such as the use of antilymphocytic leukemic serum, are also under study.[28]

Preliminary data indicate that periodic therapy with remission-inducing agents ("periodic reinduction") produces more prolonged remissions and greater longevity. It is likely that such programs will soon become standard therapy for treatment of leukemia victims.

CHEMOTHERAPY OF ACUTE MYELOCYTIC LEUKEMIA

Progress in the treatment of acute myelocytic leukemia has lagged behind progress in treating acute lymphocytic leukemia of childhood. There is no lack of agents that are effective in reducing the number of leukemic cells; see Table 10–4 and refs. 18, 25, 26,

TABLE 10-4 *Drugs Used in Treatment of Acute Myelocytic Leukemia*

AGENT	REMISSION INDUCTION RATE	COMMENT
Single agent		
6-Mercaptopurine	5–15%	Most widely used in *conventional* therapy
Methotrexate	0–50%	Used in intensive courses with high toxicity (ref. 30)
Methyl-methylglyoxalbisguanyl hydrazone	20–30%	*Experimental;* too toxic for standard use (ref. 31)
Cytosine arabinoside	15–25%	Promising *experimental* agent, especially in combination therapy (ref. 18)
Daunomycin	?	*Experimental;* toxic; ultimate use uncertain (ref. 26)
6-Methyl-mercaptopurine riboside	?	*Ineffective alone;* enhances effectiveness of 6-mercaptopurine (ref. 32)
Combinations of agents (experimental)		
6-Mercaptopurine + 6-methyl mercaptopurine riboside	?	refs. 29, 32
Daunomycin + other drugs	?	ref. 26
Cytosine arabinoside + 6-thioguanine	>20%	ref. 33
6-Mercaptopurine + methotrexate, + vincristine, + prednisone	25–60%	refs. 25, 34

29–33. Unfortunately, clinically useful cytotoxicity against the malignant cells is usually accompanied by severe toxicity to normal marrow elements. A pertinent clinical observation is that the normal blood elements do not recover after treatment of acute myelocytic leukemia in the same manner that normal elements recover after therapy of acute lymphocytic leukemia. Freireich and his colleagues[29] have suggested that virtual destruction of normal, hematopoietic cells may be required for the induction of remission in acute myelocytic leukemia.

To speak of "traditional therapy" of acute myelocytic leukemia is virtually meaningless, since treatment with agents in existence more than 5 years ago produced remissions in less than 10 per cent of the patients. We are still exploring the optimal use of new drugs and new drug combinations to treat this highly malignant disorder.

Conventional therapy has consisted of 6-mercaptopurine, 2.5 mg. per kg. per day by mouth, or 6-mercaptopurine, 1 mg. per kg. per day in combination with therapeutic doses of allopurinol (400 mg. per day). Despite the fact that under the best circumstances only 10 per cent of patients with acute myelocytic leukemia will achieve a complete hematologic remission with 6-mercaptopurine, it is still the therapy of choice when intensive supportive care cannot be given. Therefore, unless the patient is referred to a special treatment center, 6-mercaptopurine should be used.

There is still considerable controversy as to whether corticosteroids should be used in conjunction with 6-mercaptopurine.[35] Certainly steroids should never be used alone. If a patient treated with a combination of corticosteroids and 6-mercaptopurine shows evidence of accelerated disease, such as a rapidly rising white blood count or an increase in organomegaly, steroids should be discontinued promptly.

In my opinion, *all therapy other than 6-mercaptopurine is experimental and should be administered only in centers prepared to provide intensive supportive care.* With new drugs and combination therapy, remission rates have increased sharply to 25 to 30 per cent (Table 10–4). It is not clear, however, that there has been a comparable increase in longevity. Promising combinations of drugs are listed in Table 10–4.

At the present time the best results in the treatment of acute myelocytic leukemia are probably being achieved with a combination of cytosine arabinoside and thioguanine.[33] Cytosine arabinoside is not available for general use. My own experience suggests that one can achieve complete remission or very good partial remission in over 40 per cent of patients with both agents given in dosages of 2.5 mg. per kg. per day. Such therapy is often associated with transient marrow hypoplasia but few other untoward side effects. Striking megaloblastic changes in the marrow red cell precursors are the rule with adequate treatment.

We have achieved almost as high a rate of remission induction (about 30 per cent) with a modified "VAMP" program in which very high dosages of prednisolone (e.g., 1 gm. per day), methotrexate, 6-MP, and vincristine are given in an intensive 5-day course.[25] Such therapy is usually accompanied by profound toxicity. Bone marrow depression and gastrointestinal disturbances are usually temporary, but vincristine-induced neuropathy is often irreversible. Notwithstanding, we have found "VAMP" to be the best alternative to the continuation of cytosine arabinoside and thioguanine. With such programs we are, of course, prepared to offer intensive supportive therapy including, on occasion, bone marrow transplantation from a compatible donor.

GUIDELINES FOR CHEMOTHERAPY

Indications for Stopping or Modifying Treatment

Whether standard or experimental therapy is used, certain practical guidelines are necessary to determine when treatment of acute leukemia should be continued or stopped. Several parameters should be followed: the peripheral white blood cell count and the differential count; the reticulocyte and platelet counts; bone marrow morphology; the size of liver, spleen, and lymph nodes; sternal tenderness; and bone pain. Of these, *the characteristics of the peripheral blood and bone marrow are the critical guides to therapy.* It is important, therefore, to distinguish the patient with a persistently low white blood cell count and few blast cells in the peripheral blood. Such a patient is said to have aleukemic leukemia; of necessity, the bone marrow composition and not the peripheral blood is the major guide to the treatment of such a patient.

When the absolute number of blast cells in the peripheral blood and the percentage of the blast cells in the marrow aspirate are unchanged by drug therapy, either the drug is ineffective or the trial has been inadequate (less than 4 to 8 weeks). Conversely, if the number of blasts in the peripheral blood falls to low levels or disappears, then the drug is considered to be at least partially effective. When the blast cells disappear from the blood, the bone marrow becomes the principal guide to treatment. Similarly, an increase in reticulocytes, granulocytes, or platelets in the peripheral blood is usually an index of suppression of malignant cells by the cytotoxic drugs. When these normal blood elements begin to increase in number, the bone marrow becomes the guide to subsequent treatment.

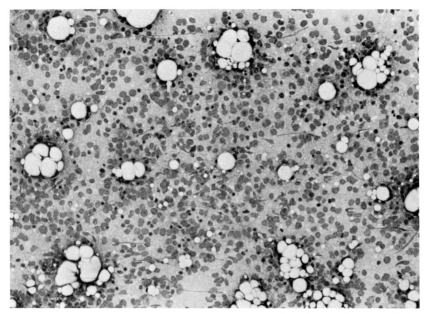

Figure 10–1 Bone marrow in patient with acute lymphocytic leukemia before chemotherapy. (Original magnification, 250 ×.)

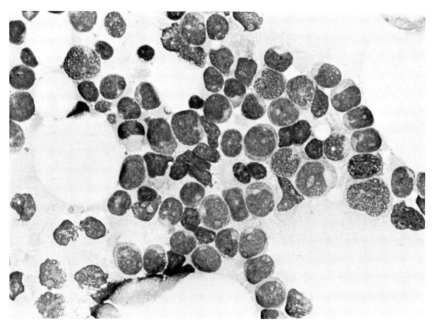

Figure 10-2 Same patient as in Figure 10-1. (Original magnification, 1250 ×.)

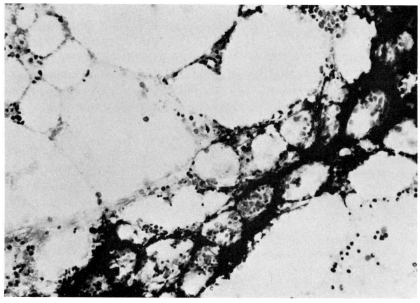

Figure 10-3 Bone marrow from the same patient with acute lymphocytic leukemia after chemotherapy. Note hypoplasia of the bone marrow. (Original magnification, 250 ×.)

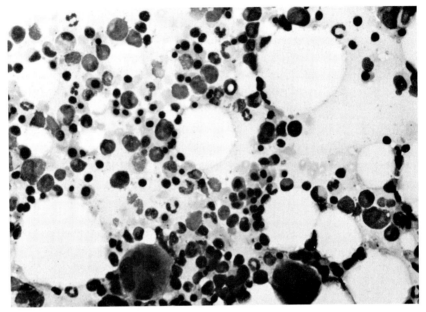

Figure 10-4 Bone marrow from the same patient with acute lymphocytic leukemia showing early recovery of hematopoietic elements. Megakaryocytes and normoblasts are evident. (Original magnification, 800 ×.)

The sequence of morphologic events in the leukemic bone marrow as a reflection of drug treatment is illustrated in Figures 10-1 to
10-4. Before treatment, the bone marrow is packed with malignant
cells (Figs. 10-1 and 10-2). The normal fat spaces are obliterated and
the morphologic picture is "deadly dull" because the marrow is
replaced by primitive cells, which are all at about the same stage of
differentiation. With effective drug therapy, the marrow becomes
hypocellular, generally with a few blast cells remaining (Fig. 10-3).
At this time, drug treatment is sharply reduced to allow the normal
marrow elements to regenerate. Regeneration is at first spotty; normal marrow elements, including megakaryocytes, appear in a slightly
hypoplastic marrow (Fig. 10-4). A small percentage of blast cells at
this stage is acceptable. As a rule, when this type of marrow is found,
treatment with "maintaining" drugs is begun.

LEUKEMIC INFILTRATION OF THE CENTRAL NERVOUS SYSTEM

As patients with acute leukemia, and in particular acute lymphoblastic leukemia, live longer, central nervous system involvement by the malignant process has become more common. The

reasons for this increase in frequency are multiple, but it is likely that the major factor resides in the properties of the drugs used in chemotherapy. Most of the cytotoxic agents used to treat leukemia do not effectively cross the blood-brain barrier. Consequently, the meninges become a privileged site for the replication of leukemic cells. Thus, the peripheral blood and bone marrow may be entirely normal by morphologic criteria (complete peripheral remission), but leukemic cells continue to proliferate in the meninges. This situation is less common in acute myeloblastic leukemia, either because of the different character of the leukemic cell or because the patients do not live long enough to develop the complications of central nervous system leukemia.

In some instances, the neurologic manifestations of central nervous system involvement may be minimal without signs or symptoms sufficient to permit anatomic localization. Some patients are incorrectly diagnosed; for example, there are patients with central nervous system leukemia who have been treated for chronic sinusitis for several weeks. Therefore, persistent headache is sufficient reason for performing a lumbar puncture to establish or rule out the diagnosis of central nervous system leukemia.

In some cases, the signs of central nervous system leukemia may be quite flagrant, with papilledema, sixth-nerve palsies, ataxia, and intractable vomiting. In children, roentgenograms of the skull may reveal diastasis of the sutures and increased digital markings if this condition has been present for a long time.

The character of the spinal fluid is usually sufficient to establish the diagnosis of central nervous system leukemic infiltration and to distinguish it from that seen in the major neurologic complications of acute leukemia—intracranial hemorrhage and infection of the central nervous system. With leukemic infiltration, the spinal fluid protein is almost always elevated, the sugar is often low, and leukemic cells are detectable.[36–38] It is mandatory that cultures for bacteria and fungi be obtained, and that India ink examination for *Cryptococcus* be performed. The leukemic character of the cells in the spinal fluid may be difficult to establish by standard cytologic techniques. Relatively simple staining procedures are available, however.[37] At one institution, an instrument called the Cytocentrifuge (Shandon Scientific Products Co.) is used to deposit the cells on a glass slide before staining with Wright's stain. The Cytocentrifuge produces uniform, well-spaced, cellular preparations with well-preserved cellular detail.

Once the diagnosis of central nervous system leukemia is established, therapy should be instituted quickly. At the present time the treatment of choice is intrathecally administered methotrexate.[36, 39, 40] Since the drug may be absorbed through the meninges and exert a systemic effect, methotrexate must be used with caution in the patient with drug-induced marrow depression or impaired renal function. Occasionally citrovorum factor is given parenterally, concomitantly with intrathecally administered methotrexate, to prevent the systemic effect of a folic acid antagonist. Another important factor is the volume in which the drug is administered. If possible, this volume should approximate 10 per cent of the spinal fluid volume, roughly 10 to 15 ml. in an adult. This volume cannot always be achieved when the spinal fluid pressure is significantly elevated.

An occasional patient will fail to respond to intrathecally administered methotrexate. In unresponsive patients, the therapeutic alternatives (in the order of the author's preference) are: (1) external irradiation of the central nervous system, (2) high-dose adrenal corticosteroids (e.g., prednisone, 120 mg. per day in an adult), and (3) experimental therapy such as intrathecally administered L-asparaginase.

Several experimental agents have been tried with some success, including BCNU[41] and L-asparaginase.[42] Central nervous system infiltration in acute myelocytic leukemia is so rare that no generally accepted treatment schedule has been devised. The few patients with central nervous system infiltration complicating acute myelocytic leukemia who have been seen at the University of California San Francisco Medical Center in recent years have all responded well to intrathecally administered methotrexate.

In acute lymphoblastic leukemia, autopsy data indicate that leukemic cell infiltration of the meninges may persist despite aggressive therapy. It is likely, therefore, that the therapy generally fails to eradicate leukemic cells permanently from the central nervous system, although it may effectively control the clinical manifestations.

ILLUSTRATIVE CASE HISTORY: ACUTE LYMPHOBLASTIC
LEUKEMIA

The clinical course of the patient is summarized in Figure 10–5. In September 1968, a 21-year-old woman consulted her physician, complaining of weakness, lethargy, and persistent lymphadenopathy following an upper respiratory infection. A diagnosis of acute lymphoblastic leukemia was made on the basis of the morphology of the peripheral blood and bone marrow. Treatment was begun with allopurinol, 400 mg. per day, prednisone, 80 mg. per day, and vincristine, 2 mg. intravenously, once weekly. Vincristine therapy was discontinued after the third dose because the patient complained of paresthesia and numbness of the fingers.

By early October 1968, the peripheral blood and bone marrow had returned to normal. The prednisone dose was gradually reduced at the same time that treatment with 6-MP, 150 mg. per day, was initiated. The patient continued taking 6-MP and felt entirely well for 6 months; in April 1969, she was again hospitalized because of increased numbers of blasts in the periph-

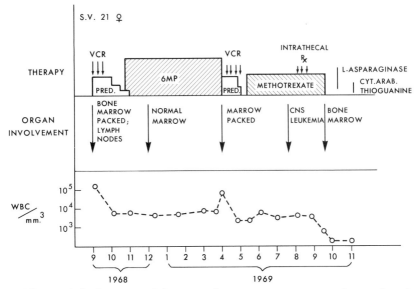

Figure 10–5 Sequence of therapy and response in a patient with acute lymphocytic leukemia. See case history.

eral blood. Remission was again induced with prednisone and a small dose
of vincristine (1 mg. per week). In order to maintain the remission, cyclic
treatment with methotrexate was initiated at doses of 5 mg. per day alternating with 10 mg. per day.

In *August 1969*, when the patient was still in complete hematologic
remission, she began to complain of severe headaches. A diagnosis of central
nervous system leukemic infiltration was made and she was given methotrexate intrathecally, with a good response. After intrathecal therapy, oral therapy was resumed.

In *September 1969*, the patient developed leukopenia and thrombocytopenia, and increased numbers of lymphoblasts appeared in the bone marrow. A relapse of her disease was diagnosed. Attempts at inducing a remission with prednisone, vincristine, and cyclophosphamide were unsuccessful.
Experimental drug protocols, first L-asparaginase and then a combination of
cytosine arabinoside and thioguanine, were used in an attempt to control her
disease. These drugs produced only temporary amelioration of her disease,
and the patient died of sepsis from gram-negative bacteria in November
1969.

COMMENT: Standard therapy was used to induce and maintain
remission of acute lymphoblastic leukemia on two occasions. During
the second remission, when the patient's blood and bone marrow
were morphologically normal, she developed leukemic infiltration of
the central nervous system. Meningeal disease responded to intrathecally administered methotrexate. When the patient's disease relapsed for the third time and failed to respond to standard agents,
experimental drugs and drug protocols were tried, without success.

Illustrative Case History: Acute Myelocytic Leukemia

The clinical course of the patient and response to therapy are shown in Figure 10-6.

The patient, 40 years of age, was asymptomatic until *August 1969*, when he noted that he became fatigued more easily than usual and began to lose weight. In early *October 1969*, he had an upper respiratory infection and fever (101° F.). His physician found axillary lymphadenopathy and petechiae of the skin and mucous membranes. The patient was admitted to a community hospital where laboratory determinations included hematocrit of 25 per cent, a white blood count of 2800 per cu. mm., with blasts in the peripheral blood, and a platelet count of 20,000 per cu. mm.; a bone marrow specimen was interpreted as acute myelocytic leukemia (Fig. 10–7).

His physician began therapy with 6-mercaptopurine and prednisone, but soon experienced difficulty in controlling bleeding from thrombocytopenia. The patient was then referred to the University of California Hospitals, San Francisco, on *October 29, 1969*.

On physical examination, pallor, ecchymoses, and splenomegaly were noted. The serum uric acid and creatinine were normal. The patient was placed in a "reverse isolation environment" and on *November 1, 1969*, therapy was initiated with allopurinol, 400 mg. daily; cytosine arabinoside, 2 mg. per kg. daily by rapid intravenous injection; and 6-thioguanine, 1.5 mg. per kg. daily by mouth. Supportive therapy with packed red blood cells and platelets was given as needed. Repeated bone marrow aspirations were performed to serve as a guide to response to therapy.

By *November 17, 1969* (day 17 of treatment), there was a marked decrease

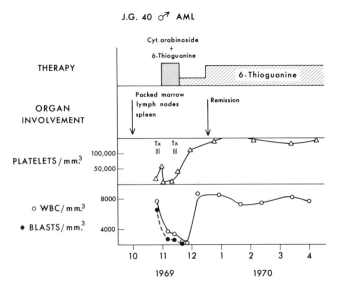

Figure 10–6 Sequence of therapy and response in a patient with acute myelocytic leukemia. See case history.

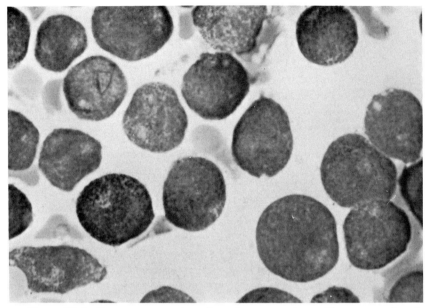

Figure 10–7 Bone marrow aspirate from the same patient with acute myelocytic leukemia as in Figure 10–6, in relapse. (Original magnification, 1250 ×.)

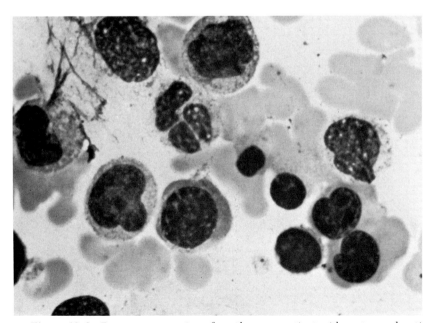

Figure 10–8 Bone marrow aspirate from the same patient with acute myelocytic leukemia as in Figures 10–6 and 10–7, after drug-induced remission. Increased numbers of normoblasts are apparent. (Original magnification, 1250 ×.)

in marrow cellularity. At this time cytosine arabinoside was discontinued and maintenance therapy with 6-thioguanine at a reduced dosage (0.75 mg. per kg. daily by mouth) was initiated. The peripheral white blood count was then 700 per cu. mm. and the platelet count before transfusion ranged from 10,000 to 14,000 per cu. mm. The patient had a brief episode of bacterial infection, which responded readily to antibiotic therapy. By *November 25, 1969*, there was clear evidence of bone marrow recovery and the peripheral platelet count had risen to 125,000 per cu. mm. When the patient was discharged from the hospital on *December 1, 1969*, he was receiving 6-thioguanine as his only medication. The marrow at that time showed complete remission of the disease; focal erythroid hyperplasia was the only abnormal finding (Fig. 10–8).

The patient has remained in remission until the present time and takes 6-thioguanine, 2 mg. per kg. daily by mouth.

COMMENT: This patient with acute myelocytic leukemia was referred to a special treatment center when the difficulties of providing adequate supportive care in the community hospital became too great. An excellent remission was achieved and is still being maintained with an experimental drug protocol consisting of cytosine arabinoside and 6-thioguanine.

REFERENCES

1. Skipper, H. E., Schnabel, F. M., Jr., and Wilcox, W. S.: Experimental evaluation of potential anti-cancer agents. XIV. Cancer Chemother. Rep., *45*:5, 1965.
2. Skipper, H. E.: Biochemical, biological, pharmacologic, toxicologic, kinetic, and clinical (subhuman and human) relationships. Cancer, *21*:600, 1968.
3. Zubrod, C. G.: Treatment of acute leukemias. Cancer Res., *27*:2557, 1967.
4. Cutler, S. J., Axtell, L., and Heise, H.: Ten thousand cases of leukemia: 1940–62. J. Nat. Cancer Inst., *39*:993, 1967.
5. Dameshek, W., and Gunz, F.: Leukemia. Ed. 2. New York, Grune & Stratton, Inc., 1964.
6. Boggs, D. R., Wintrobe, M. M., and Cartwright, G. E.: The acute leukemias: Analysis of 322 cases and review of the literature. Medicine, *41*:163, 1962.
7. Frei, E., III, and Freireich, E. J.: Progress and perspective in the chemotherapy of acute leukemia. Advances Chemother., *2*:269, 1965.
8. Frei, E., III: Chemotherapy of acute leukemia. *In* Brodsky, I., Kahn, S. B., and Moyer, J. H. (Editors): Cancer Chemotherapy. New York, Grune & Stratton, Inc., 1967, p. 185.
9. Leikin, S. L., Brubaker, C., Hartmann, J. R., Murphy, M. L., Wolff, J. A., and Perrin, E.: Varying prednisone dosage in remission induction of previously untreated childhood leukemia. Cancer, *21*:346–351, 1968.
10. Krivit, W., Brubaker, C., Thatcher, L. G., Pierce, M., Perrin, E., and Hartmann, J. R.: Maintenance therapy in acute leukemia of childhood. Comparison of cyclic vs. sequential methods. Cancer, *21*:352–356, 1968.
11. Farber, S., Diamond, L. K., Mercer, R. D., Sylvester, R. F., Jr., and Wolff, J. A.: Temporary remission in acute leukemia in children produced by folic acid antagonist 4-amino-pteroyl glutamic acid (aminopterin). New Eng. J. Med., *238*:787, 1948.
12. New treatment schedule with improved survival in childhood leukemia. Acute leukemia Group B. J.A.M.A., *194*:75, 1965.
13. Djerassi, I., Royer, G., Treat, C., and Abir, E.: Survival of children with acute

lymphatic leukemia—role of methotrexate and intensive supportive management. Proc. Amer. Assoc. Cancer Res., 8:14, 1967.

14. Farber, S.: Chemotherapy in the treatment of leukemia and Wilms' tumor. J.A.M.A., 198:826, 1966.

15. Haggard, M. E.: Vincristine (NSC 67574) therapy for acute leukemia in children. Cancer Chemother. Rep., 52:477, 1968.

16. Evans, A. E.: Vincristine (NSC 67574) in the treatment of children with acute leukemia. Cancer Chemother. Rep., 52:469, 1968.

17. Fernbach, D. J., Sutow, W. W., Thurman, W. G., and Vietti, T. J.: Clinical evaluation of cyclophosphamide, a new agent for the treatment of children with acute leukemia. J.A.M.A., 182:30, 1962.

18. Ellison, R. R., et al.: Arabinosyl cytosine: A useful agent in the treatment of acute leukemia in adults. Blood, 32:507–523, 1968.

19. Holton, C. P., Lonsdale, D., Nora, A. H., Thurman, W. G., and Vietti, T. J.: Clinical study of daunomycin (NCS-82151) in children with acute leukemia. Cancer, 22:1014–1017, 1968.

20. Lessner, H. E., et al.: BCNU (1,3, bis (β-chloroethyl)-1-nitrosourea). Effects on advanced Hodgkin's disease and other neoplasia. Cancer, 22:451–456, 1968.

21. Oettgen, H. F., et al.: Inhibition of leukemias in man by L-asparaginase. Cancer Res., 27:2619, 1967.

22. Cline, M. J.: Acute leukemia. Current concepts of pathogenesis and treatment. California Med., 109:146, 1968.

23. Zubrod, C. G.: New developments in the chemotherapy of the leukemias and lymphomas. In Jaffe, E. R. (editor): Plenary Session Papers, XII Congress, International Society of Hematology. New York, 1968, p. 32.

24. Djerassi, I.: Methotrexate infusions and intensive supportive care in the management of children with acute lymphocytic leukemia: Follow-up report. Cancer Res., 27:2561, 1967.

25. Henderson, E. S.: Combination chemotherapy of acute lymphocytic leukemia of childhood. Cancer Res., 27:2570, 1967.

26. Bernard, J.: Acute leukemia treatment. Cancer Res., 27:2565, 1967.

27. Mathe, G., et al.: Acute lymphoblastic leukemia treated with a combination of prednisone, vincristine, and rubidomycin. Lancet, 2:380, 1967.

28. Miller, D. G., Moldovanu, G., Kaplan, A., and Tocci, S.: Antilymphocytic leukemic serum and chemotherapy in the treatment of murine leukemia. Cancer, 22:1191–1198, 1968.

29. Freireich, E. J., Bodey, G. P., Harris, J. E., and Hart, J. S.: Therapy for acute granulocytic leukemia. Cancer Res., 27:2573, 1967.

30. Huguley, C. M., Jr., Vogler, W. R., Lea, J. W., Corely, C. C., and Lowrey, M. E.: Acute leukemia treated with divided doses of methotrexate. Arch. Intern. Med., 115:23, 1965.

31. Levin, R. H., Henderson, E., Karon, M., and Freireich, E. J.: Treatment of acute leukemia with methylglyoxal-bis-guanylhydrazone (methyl GAG). Clin. Pharm. Ther., 6:31, 1965.

32. Luce, J. K., Samuels, M. L., and Freireich, E. J.: The effect of schedule and dose on toxicity and antileukemic activity of 6-methyl-mercaptopurine riboside (NSC 40774). Proc. Amer. Assoc. Cancer Res., 8:42, 1967.

33. Gee, T. S., et al.: Combination therapy of adult acute leukemia with thioguanine (TG) and 1-beta-D-arabinofuranosyl cytosine (CA). Proc. Amer. Assoc. Cancer Res., 9:23, 1968.

34. Karon, M., Freireich, E. J., and Carbone, P.: Effective combination therapy of adult acute leukemia. Proc. Amer. Assoc. Cancer Res., 6:34, 1965.

35. Krospe, W. H., and Conrad, M. E.: The danger of corticosteroids in acute granulocytic leukemia. Med. Clin. N. Amer., 50:1653, 1966.

36. Nieri, R. L., Burgert, E. O., Jr., and Groover, R. V.: Central-nervous-system complications of leukemia: A review. Proc. Mayo Clin., 43:70–79, 1968.

37. Nies, B. A., Malmgren, R. A., Chu, E. W., Del Vecchio, P. R., Thomas, L. B., and Freireich, E. J.: Cerebrospinal fluid cytology in patients with acute leukemia. Cancer, 18:1385, 1965.

38. Skeel, R. T., Yankee, R. A., and Henderson, E. S.: Meningeal leukemia. J.A.M.A., 205:155, 1968.

39. Evans, A. E., D'Angio, G. J., and Mitus, A.: Central nervous system complications of children with acute leukemia. An evaluation of treatment methods. J. Pediat., 64:94, 1964.
40. Hyman, C. B., Bogle, J. M., Brubaker, C. A., Williams, K., and Hammond, D.: Central nervous system involvement by leukemia in children. II. Therapy with intrathecal methotrexate. Blood, 25:13–22, 1965.
41. Rall, D. P.: Experimental studies of the blood-brain barrier. Cancer Res., 25: 1752, 1965.
42. Tan, C., and Oettgen, H.: Clinical experience with L-asparaginase administered intrathecally. Proc. Amer. Assoc. Cancer Res., 10:92, 1969.

Recent Additional Bibliography Not Cited in Text

43. Burchenal, J. H.: Success and failure in present chemotherapy and the implications of asparaginase. Cancer Res., 29:2262–2269, 1969.
44. Hart, J. S., Shirakawa, S., Trujillo, J., and Frei, E., III: The mechanism of induction of complete remission in acute myeloblastic leukemia in man. Cancer Res., 29:2300–2307, 1969.
45. Leikin, S., Brubaker, C., Hartmann, J., Murphy, M. L., and Wolff, J.: The use of combination therapy in leukemia remission. Cancer, 24:427–432, 1969.
46. Lampkin, B. C., Nagao, T., and Mauer, A. M.: Synchronization of the mitotic cycle in acute leukemia. Nature, 222:1274–1275, 1969.
47. Hryniuk, W. M., and Bertino, J. R.: Treatment of leukemia with large doses of methotrexate and folinic acid: Clinical-biochemical correlates. J. Clin. Invest., 48:2140–2155, 1969.
48. Burchenal, J. H., and Karnofsky, D. A.: Clinical evaluation of L-asparaginase. Introduction. Cancer, 25:241–243, 1970.
49. Oettgen, H. F., Stephenson, P. A., Schwartz, M. K., Leeper, R. D., Tallal, L., Tan, C. C., Clarkson, B. D., Golbey, R. B., Krakoff, I. H., Karnofsky, D. A., Murphy, M. L., and Burchenal, J. H.: Toxicity of E. coli L-asparaginase in man. Cancer, 25:253–278, 1970.
50. Tallal, L., Tan, C., Oettgen, H., Wollner, N., McCarthy, M., Helson, L., Burchenal, J. Karnofsky, D., and Murphy, M. L.: E. coli L-asparaginase in the treatment of leukemia and solid tumors in 131 children. Cancer, 25:306–320, 1970.
51. Wang, J. J., Selawry, O. S., Vietti, T. J., and Bodey, G. P., Sr.: Prolonged infusion of arabinosyl cytosine in childhood leukemia. Cancer, 25:1–6, 1970.
52. Nagao, T., Lampkin, B. C., and Mauer, A. M.: Maintenance therapy in acute childhood leukemia. J. Pediat., 76:134–137, 1970.
53. Sullivan, M. P., Vietti, T. J., Fernbach, D. J., Griffith, K. M., Haddy, T. B., and Watkins, W. L.: Clinical investigations in the treatment of meningeal leukemia: Radiation therapy regimens vs. conventional intrathecal methotrexate. Blood, 34:301–319, 1969.
54. Wang, J. J., and Pratt, C. B.: Intrathecal arabinosyl cytosine in meningeal leukemia. Cancer, 25:531–534, 1970.

CHAPTER 11

CHRONIC LEUKEMIA

CHRONIC MYELOCYTIC LEUKEMIA

Clinical Manifestations and Diagnosis

In any discussion of the treatment of chronic myelocytic leukemia (chronic granulocytic leukemia), a few words regarding diagnosis and natural history are appropriate.

The clinical distinctions between chronic myelocytic leukemia and a leukemoid reaction are not universally appreciated. Granulocytic leukocytosis resulting from inflammatory disease or associated with certain solid tumors is a leukemoid reaction. Both chronic myelocytic leukemia and leukemoid reactions may be characterized by very high levels of circulating granulocytes (in excess of 100,000 per cu. mm.), immaturity of the granulocytes in the peripheral blood, hyperplastic bone marrow that is predominantly granulocytic with a preponderance of young forms ("shift to the left"), increased serum uric acid, and hepatosplenomegaly. The morphologic appearance of peripheral blood and bone marrow is insufficient to distinguish between chronic myelocytic leukemia and a leukemoid reaction. The bone marrow picture may be consistent with chronic myelocytic leukemia, but it is never diagnostic. Clinical features suggesting chronic myelocytic leukemia are absolute basophilia of the peripheral blood, thrombocytosis, and large numbers of megakaryocytes in the bone marrow aspirate.

Two tests are useful in establishing the diagnosis of chronic myelocytic leukemia: determination of the leukocyte alkaline phosphatase level and analysis of the karyotype of the blood cells. The leukocyte alkaline phosphatase value is generally high in leukemoid reactions; it is almost always low in patients with chronic myelocytic

137

leukemia in relapse. The leukocyte alkaline phosphatase level is often low in several other diseases: infectious mononucleosis, idiopathic thrombocytopenic purpura, and paroxysmal nocturnal hemoglobinuria. However, there is little in the clinical manifestations of these diseases to cause confusion with chronic myelocytic leukemia. The only disorder that may clinically resemble chronic myelocytic leukemia and in which the leukocyte alkaline phosphatase is occasionally low is agnogenic myeloid metaplasia. A bone marrow biopsy serves to distinguish these diseases, revealing increased fibrotic tissue in myeloid metaplasia.

The bone marrow contains the typical Philadelphia abnormality of the chromosomes in almost 90 per cent of patients with chronic myelocytic leukemia.[1] This abnormality can also be demonstrated in the peripheral blood when there are circulating immature granulocytes. The Philadelphia chromosome appears to be pathognomonic for chronic myelocytic leukemia and has not been demonstrated in any other disease except for a few cases of acute leukemia.[2] Roughly 10 per cent of the patients with chronic myelocytic leukemia are said to be Philadelphia chromosome-negative. Such patients may have an atypical and more aggressive disease that is less responsive to therapy.[1]

Chronic myelocytic leukemia can occur in any age group, although it is most common in middle age. The initial clinical features are usually anemia, symptomatic splenomegaly, weight loss, night sweats, and occasionally bleeding. In general, the level of the white blood count, the size of the spleen, and severity of clinical symptomatology tend to vary concomitantly. In contrast to the patient with chronic lymphocytic leukemia, the patient with chronic myelocytic leukemia is rarely asymptomatic when the white blood count exceeds 50,000 per cu. mm.

Patients with chronic myelocytic leukemia survive, on the average, 3 to 4 years from the time of diagnosis. With good management, the patient is often symptom free until the terminal manifestations of disease. Probably the most common preterminal event is a transition to a disease that is indistinguishable from acute myelocytic leukemia, blast crisis. When blast crisis occurs, more primitive cells appear in the marrow and peripheral blood, the Philadelphia chromosome may persist or disappear, and other chromosomal abnormalities can be detected. A small percentage of patients die from complications of their disease before the appearance of blast crisis. Thrombocytopenia and bleeding may result from the basic disease or from treatment. Occasionally too vigorous therapy results in aplastic marrow, granulocytopenia, and complications such as infections. A few patients develop a disease picture resembling myeloid metaplasia, including fibrotic marrow. Chronic myelocytic leukemia in infants and children appears to have a different natural history from that in adults. The prognosis of the so-called juvenile type of chronic myelo-cytic leukemia is poor.[3, 4]

Objectives of Therapy

The available modalities of treatment of chronic myelocytic leukemia probably do not significantly prolong life. There is no question, however, that treatment makes the patient more comfortable and improves his capacity to function; therefore, the objective of treatment is to maintain the patient symptom free for as long a period as possible without risking complications arising from therapy.

Because there is a parallelism between symptom status and the degree of peripheral blood granulocytosis, the level of the white blood count is used as a guide to treatment. Simply stated, *therapy is directed toward maintaining the white blood count at or near the normal level.*

Modes of Therapy

Two types of treatment have proved effective in chronic myelo-cytic leukemia: splenic irradiation and chemotherapy. A number of drugs effectively reduce the level of the white blood count, includ-ing alkylators, 6-mercaptopurine, colcemide, trimethylcolchicinic acid, hydroxyurea,[5] dibromomannitol,[6] and daunomycin;[7] however, only the first two of these have had widespread clinical use. The most widely used drug is busulfan (Myleran). In the occasional patient who is unresponsive to busulfan, 6-mercaptopurine is the alternative drug of choice.

Busulfan is available in 2 mg. tablets. It is given by mouth, in a dosage of 6 to 8 mg. per day for adults, until the white blood count reaches approximately 20,000 per cu. mm. At that time, the dosage is reduced by half and the drug is continued until the white blood count reaches 10,000 to 12,000 per cu. mm., when the drug is discontinued. Busulfan therapy is not resumed until the white count rises above approximately 15,000 per cu. mm. The lowest dosage that will keep the white blood count at about 10,000 per cu. mm. is used for main-tenance therapy.[8] A careful watch is kept on the platelet count during treatment, since it may sometimes fall abruptly. Induction of the normal hematologic status may take 3 to 6 weeks, and occasionally longer. (The hematopoietic toxicity and side effects of busulfan therapy, including pulmonary fibrosis, skin pigmentation, and a syndrome resembling Addison's disease, are discussed in Chapter 2.)

Occasional patients have disease that is refractory to treatment with busulfan.[8] Such patients can be treated with 6-mercaptopurine.[9] This drug is somewhat more difficult to use than busulfan in the treatment of chronic myelocytic leukemia: control with 6-mercaptopurine is not as smooth, and unpredictable thrombocytopenia may occur. The usual dosage of 6-mercaptopurine is 2 to 2.5 mg. per kg. per day by mouth. The dosage is reduced to one-third of this level if allopurinol is used concomitantly to control hyperuricemia.

An often neglected observation is that splenic irradiation is approximately as effective as busulfan in the treatment of chronic myelocytic leukemia. Small doses of 200 to 600 rads in 7 to 10 days can produce a striking decrease in the size of the spleen, a concomitant fall in the peripheral white blood count, and a return of the bone marrow to a morphologically normal status.[10] Such a remission may last for many months and occasionally years. When subsequent relapses occur, the patient can again be given a course of radiation therapy, although it is usually less effective than the initial course.

For the sake of completeness, it should be noted that a few clinics still use radioactive phosphorus in the treatment of chronic myelocytic leukemia.[11] There is insufficient evidence to recommend this form of therapy as being superior to drug treatment.

Remissions induced by either drugs or irradiation are associated with the return of the leukocyte alkaline phosphatase to normal, but persistence of the Philadelphia chromosome in the marrow.

Unless the patient dies of complications of his disease or of therapy, the clinical picture of blast crisis usually supervenes. The characteristics of this terminal phase have recently been reviewed and resemble those of acute myelocytic leukemia.[12] Blast crisis is treated in the same way as acute myelocytic leukemia (Chapter 10). Busulfan and splenic irradiation are of no value during this phase of the disease.

Zubrod[13] has reviewed recent developments in the treatment of chronic myelocytic leukemia and has stated, "The slower pace of the chronic leukemias has led to this curious situation: Even though these diseases are 100 per cent fatal, physicians have chosen to treat symptoms rather than use the available drugs (plus x-irradiation) in an attempt to eradicate the leukemic cells." He has thus succinctly summarized the existing situation in regard to the treatment of chronic myelocytic leukemia. It is to be hoped that in the future a more vigorous approach may be used in the treatment of this uniformly fatal disease.

ILLUSTRATIVE CASE HISTORY: CHRONIC MYELOCYTIC LEUKEMIA

The patient's clinical course is summarized in Figure 11-1.

In *February 1966*, a 45-year-old man consulted his physician because of weakness and exertional dyspnea. He was found to be severely anemic and to have a white blood count greater than 100,000 per cu. mm. He was referred to the University of California Hospitals, San Francisco, with a probable diagnosis of chronic myelocytic leukemia. The diagnosis was confirmed by the findings of the typical Philadelphia chromosome in the blood and bone marrow and a low white blood cell alkaline phosphatase level. His bone marrow was packed with granulocyte precursors in all stages of maturation, and hepatosplenomegaly was present. The peripheral white blood count was 180,000 per cu. mm. with 5 per cent myeloblasts and promyelocytes and 23 per cent more mature granulocytes (Fig. 11-2). The platelet count was 1,000,000 per cu. mm. Treatment with busulfan, 6 mg. per day, was initiated. The white blood count fell rapidly and within 4 weeks it reached normal levels. The spleen decreased in size more slowly. The patient was followed thereafter for 20 months. Busulfan was adjusted to keep the peripheral white count in the range of 5000 to 15,000 per cu. mm. The patient was asymptomatic during this interval.

In *August 1967*, the patient moved to a new location and was no longer followed at our medical center. In May of 1968, 9 months later, he became severely ill and was seen once again. He was extremely anemic (hemoglobin 4 gm. per 100 ml.), he had marked hepatosplenomegaly, and his peripheral white count was 250,000 per cu mm. The serum uric acid level was 10 mg. per 100 ml. Allopurinol therapy was begun and a high fluid intake encouraged. A program of splenic irradiation was then initiated and a remission was rapidly induced. Thereafter, busulfan was resumed in doses adequate to control the peripheral white count and symptomatology. Therapy was successful until *March 1969*, when increasing numbers of myeloblasts appeared in the peripheral blood and bone marrow. A diagnosis of "blast crisis" was made and therapy with 6-MP and vincristine was introduced. The patient died 8 weeks later.

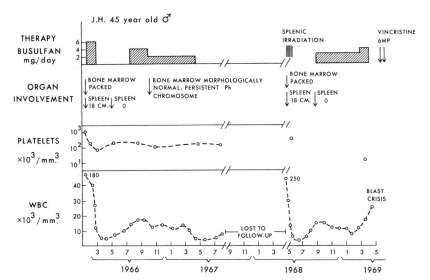

Figure 11-1 The sequence of therapy and response in a patient with chronic myelocytic leukemia. See case history.

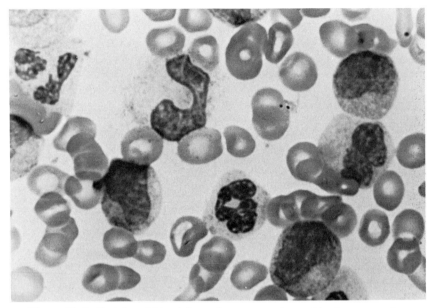

Figure 11-2 Peripheral blood from the same patient with chronic myelocytic leukemia as in Figure 11–1. See case history. (Original magnification, 1250×.)

COMMENT: The patient's disease was controlled with busulfan for several years, and he was free of symptoms. The peripheral white count was used as a guide to treatment. When the disease relapsed because of his failure to take medication, splenic irradiation rapidly induced a remission. The terminal phase of the disease resembled acute myelocytic leukemia and was unresponsive to busulfan therapy.

CHRONIC LYMPHOCYTIC LEUKEMIA

Clinical Manifestations and Diagnosis

The median survival of patients with chronic lymphocytic leukemia is 4 to 6 years from the time of diagnosis.[14, 15] Survival from the time initial symptoms appear is even longer. It is probable that many, if not the majority, of patients with chronic lymphocytic leukemia have the characteristic abnormalities in their blood and marrow for long periods of time before symptoms appear or the diagnosis is made. It is not uncommon for the abnormality to be detected first on a routine blood examination.

The characteristic leukocytosis of the peripheral blood and infiltration of the bone marrow with mature lymphocytes occur in few disorders other than chronic lymphocytic leukemia. In lymphosarcoma, the morphologic features of blood and bone marrow may be similar to those in chronic lymphocytic leukemia, but the mode of presentation and more aggressive course of lymphosarcoma usually serve to distinguish this disease entity.[16] Infectious lymphocytosis is also a disease characterized by increased numbers of lymphocytes in peripheral blood. It is usually a disease of children, occurring sporadically or in small clusters of patients, and is probably the result of infection with an enterovirus.[17] A benign course is characteristic.[18] Chronic lymphocytic leukemia is almost always a disease of adult life, although rare cases in children have been reported.[19] The disease may have a somewhat more aggressive course in the young than in the old.[15] Chronic lymphocytic leukemia is usually characterized by an unremitting albeit slowly progressive course. Spontaneous remissions have been documented only rarely.[20]

OBJECTIVES OF THERAPY

Complete hematologic remissions are very rare in chronic lymphocytic leukemia. Remission is not the objective of therapy.

The present forms of therapy do not prolong life to any significant degree.[15] Many untreated patients have a benign clinical course.[21] Therefore, treatment is directed at improving the quality of survival by treating the complications of leukemia. The major complications are as follows:

1. Collections of lymphoid tissue producing obstruction, discomfort, or disfigurement.
2. Debilitating systemic symptoms (anorexia, weight loss, night sweats).
3. Symptomatic hemolytic anemia.
4. Symptomatic thrombocytopenia.
5. Recurrent infections secondary to granulocytopenia and impaired immunologic response.

It is important to note that in chronic lymphocytic leukemia there is no correlation between the level of the white blood count and symptomatic disease. The size of the spleen and lymph nodes and complicating anemia or infection are not consistently related to the numbers of circulating white blood cells. Lymphocyte concentrations of 100,000 per cu. mm. or more may be tolerated without unusual symptoms. There is no good evidence that therapy designed to suppress lymphopoiesis prevents or delays complications. Therefore, the *white blood count is not used as a guide to therapy in chronic lymphocytic leukemia*. This is in contrast to therapy of the myelocytic form of chronic leukemia; in chronic myelocytic leukemia suppression of granulopoiesis almost always produces clinical improvement and the white blood count is used as a guide to therapy.

MODES OF THERAPY

The modalities of therapy available to the patient with chronic lymphocytic leukemia include alkylating agents,[22] adrenocorticosteroids,[23] external irradiation,[24] or internal irradiation from radioisotopes.[25]

Because treatment is directed toward alleviating the symptomatic complications of disease rather than eradication of the neoplastic cell, it is appropriate to consider the approach to each of the major complications of chronic lymphocytic leukemia.

Masses of Lymphoid Tissue Producing Obstruction, Discomfort, or Disfigurement

When such masses of lymphoid tissue are localized, they are often best treated by local radiation therapy. When they are very large, or when symptomatic lymphadenopathy is generalized, radiation therapy may be impractical, and chemotherapy should be used.

The most extensively used chemotherapeutic agent in chronic lymphocytic leukemia has been chlorambucil. This drug is generally easier to use than the other orally effective alkylators. The usual dose of chlorambucil for control of symptomatic disease is 4 to 6 mg. per day. When control of the complication has been achieved, the dose may be reduced to maintain the desired clinical effect.

A not infrequent problem facing the physician is how to treat the patient with chronic lymphocytic leukemia who has symptomatic lymphadenopathy and who also has severe thrombocytopenia or granulocytopenia, or both. In most cases, this clinical constellation is associated with bone marrow densely infiltrated with lymphocytes. In this situation, two principal therapeutic alternatives are available: a cautious trial with chlorambucil or treatment with adrenocorticosteroids. Unfortunately, no well-defined body of evidence is available as a guide to making a decision between these alternatives. My own preference is for an initial trial with prednisone, 40 to 60 mg. per day. Prednisone has a lymphocytolytic effect without myelosuppressive action;[26] however, all the risks of steroid therapy, and especially enhanced susceptibility to infection, pertain to the patient with chronic lymphocytic leukemia. In addition, the cytolytic effects of the steroid are generally transient; therefore, unless the desired lymphocytolytic effect is achieved within 4 to 6 weeks, steroids should not be continued. If the desired effect is achieved, it is desirable to stop administration of steroids as soon as possible. The physician using steroids should be forewarned that the peripheral lymphocyte count usually increases with this therapy and occasionally reaches very high levels.[23] Peripheral blood lymphocytosis occurs at a time when the lymph nodes and spleen may be shrinking; therefore, the rise in white blood count is not a contraindication to continued therapy.

Systemic Symptoms—Anorexia, Weight Loss, and Night Sweats

This constellation of symptoms—often associated with anemia—occurs sometime during the course of disease in a significant fraction of patients with chronic lymphocytic leukemia. The body burden of lymphoid tissue may be related to these symptoms, although it is not possible to document this impression. The therapeutic approach to systemic symptoms is the same as to symptomatic lymphadenopathy: chlorambucil is the first choice. Prednisone or a cautious trial with an alkylator may be used in the patient with packed marrow and significant thrombocytopenia. Rarely splenic irradiation may be helpful. When the anemia is myelophthisic rather than clearly hemolytic, androgen therapy may be beneficial.[27]

Symptomatic Hemolytic Anemia or Thrombocytopenia

These complications of chronic lymphocytic leukemia are fairly frequent and should be treated promptly. They occasionally occur after radiation therapy or chemotherapy. These complications constitute a clear-cut indication for corticosteroid therapy, to which they usually respond favorably.[23] It is often difficult, however, to discontinue steroids completely once patients have been treated for hemolytic anemia or thrombocytopenia. An attempt should be made to reduce the dose to the lowest level necessary to maintain the patient symptom-free.

Recurrent Infections

Propensity to bacteriologic infections is a complex problem resulting from either granulocytopenia or impaired immunologic response, or a combination of the two. The genesis of the defective immunologic response is not clear. Abnormalities of lymphocyte function are detectable in leukocytes from patients with chronic lymphocytic leukemia in a variety of in vitro systems.[28] It is clear, however, that the defective immunologic response involves both production of circulating antibodies and delayed hypersensitivity reactions to new antigens (primary response). Hypersensitivity reactions to previously encountered antigens remain intact.[29] The immunologic defect and granulocytopenia are reflected in an increased incidence of severe bacteriologic infections.[30] The propensity to develop severe viral infections probably results from the immunologic impairment,[31] but defective production of interferon has not been excluded as a cause of these infections. Patients with chronic lymphocytic leukemia should not be vaccinated with preparations containing living virus. Progressive vaccina after smallpox inoculation is not uncommon in these immunologically deficient patients.

The treatment of the patient with chronic lymphocytic leukemia who is prone to recurrent severe infections is one of the more vexing problems in hematology. If granulocytopenia is a contributing factor, cautious trials of chlorambucil or prednisone may be considered, although these are not effective in most patients. Occasional patients respond to treatment with androgens.

When granulocytopenia is not present and an immunologic deficiency is suspected or proved, prophylactic treatment with gamma globulin should be used. Although the effectiveness of prophylactic gamma globulin in preventing infections has not been proved by a clear-cut, double-blind study, it makes good sense to administer this relatively harmless (if painful) therapy to the infection-prone patient with chronic lymphocytic leukemia.

Because of the kinetics of gamma globulin turnover, when used therapeutically commercial gamma globulin must be given in considerable quantity, at least 30 to 40 ml. per month. Arguments have been raised that commercial gamma globulin is poor in immunoglobulin A (IgA) and that fresh-frozen plasma is a more logical replacement therapy; however, all too often plasma is a source of serum hepatitis and probably should not be used in patients who are likely to have impaired defenses against viral agents.

It is unfortunate that new and innovative approaches to the treatment of chronic lymphocytic leukemia are rare.[13] Extracorporeal irradiation of the blood[32] and the use of antilymphocyte serum[33] are interesting as scientific exercises, but appear to hold little promise for therapy in the future.

ILLUSTRATIVE CASE HISTORY: CHRONIC LYMPHOCYTIC LEUKEMIA

The patient's clinical course is summarized in Figure 11-3.

A 45-year-old man consulted his physician in *July 1966* because of purpura following minor trauma. He was found to have a white blood count of 70,000 per cu. mm. and a platelet count of 46,000 per cu. mm. The patient was referred to the University of California Hospitals, San Francisco, with a diagnosis of chronic lymphocytic leukemia.

On physical examination, pea-sized axillary and inguinal lymph nodes were palpable. The skin had numerous small ecchymoses, and a few pete-

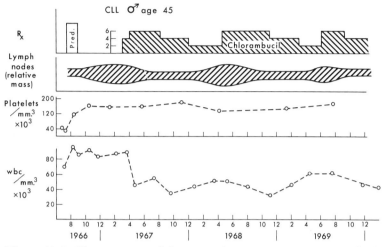

Figure 11-3 The sequence of therapy and response in a patient with chronic lymphocytic leukemia. See case history.

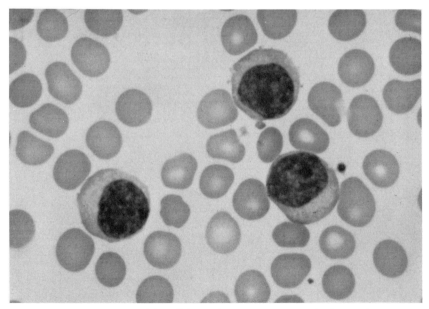

Figure 11-4 Peripheral blood from the same patient with chronic lymphocytic leukemia as in Figure 11-3. See case history. (Original magnification, 1250 ×.)

chiae were observed on the soft palate. The liver edge was felt 4 cm. below the right costal margin, but the spleen was not palpable. The white blood count was 74,000 per cu. mm. with 94 per cent mature lymphocytes (Fig. 11-4). Platelet counts varied between 36,000 and 48,000 per cu. mm. The hematocrit was normal, as were all studies of coagulation except those dependent on adequate numbers of platelets.

Treatment with prednisone, 45 mg. per day, was given over a 3-week period; the dose was then gradually reduced and discontinued entirely after 5 weeks. During this time the platelet count rose to the normal level and the white blood count to 98,000 per cu. mm. After discontinuation of steroids, the platelet count remained normal and the white blood count was in the range of 82,000 to 90,000 per cu. mm.

Thereafter, the patient was asymptomatic and received no treatment for 7 months; during this 7-month period, walnut-sized lymph nodes appeared in the submandibular and supraclavicular regions, as well as a mass (3 by 4 cm.) in the left axilla.

In *March 1967* treatment with chlorambucil, 4 mg. per day, was begun. When there was no response after 4 weeks this dose was increased to 6 mg. per day. By the sixth week, the palpable lymph nodes had shrunk to half their original size and the white blood count had fallen to 44,000 per cu. mm. The absolute number of granulocytes in the peripheral blood was unchanged.

During the subsequent year, the patient continued to take chlorambucil in doses varying between 2 and 6 mg. per day. The dose was varied according to the size of the lymph node masses, particularly those in the cervical regions that caused discomfort or were unsightly.

In *April 1968*, when the patient was taking 2 mg. of chlorambucil, he complained of generalized increase in lymphadenopathy, of weight loss, and night sweats. The symptoms disappeared after the dose of chlorambucil was increased to 6 mg. per day.

Over the subsequent two years the patient remained asymptomatic while taking chlorambucil in doses varying between 2 and 6 mg. per day. The white blood count ranged between 31,000 and 63,000 per cu mm, with about 5 per cent granulocytes. Thrombocytopenia has not recurred, and there has been no enhanced susceptibility to infection.

COMMENTS: Symptomatic thrombocytopenia was the presenting manifestation of chronic lymphocytic leukemia in this patient. The thrombocytopenia responded readily to prednisone treatment, and this steroid could eventually be discontinued. The patient was treated for three years with small doses of chlorambucil, which kept his disease under control and prevented systemic symptoms and local discomfort from lymph node masses.

REFERENCES

1. Whang-Peng, J., Canellos, G. P., Carbone, P. P., and Tjio, J. H.: Clinical implications of cytogenetic variants in chronic myelocytic leukemia (CML). Blood, 32:755–766, 1968.

2. Mastrangelo, R., Zuelzer, W., and Thompson, R. L.: The significance of the Ph[1] chromosome in acute myeloblastic leukemia: Serial cytogenetic studies in a critical case. Pediatrics, 40:834–841, 1967.
3. Hardisty, R. M., Speed, D. E., and Till, M.: Granulocytic leukemia in childhood. Brit. J. Haemat., 10:551–566, 1964.
4. Reisman, L. E., and Trujillo, J. M.: Chronic granulocytic leukemia of childhood. J. Pediat., 62:710, 1963.
5. Fishbein, W. N., Carbone, P. P., Freireich, E. J., Misra, D., and Frei, E., III: Clinical trials of hydroxyurea in patients with cancer and leukemia. Clin. Pharmacol. Ther., 5:574–580, 1964.
6. Casazza, A. R., Cahn, E. L., and Carbone, P. P.: Preliminary studies with dibromomannitol (NSC-94100) in patients with chronic myelogenous leukemia. Cancer Chemother. Rep., 51:91–97, 1967.
7. Tanzer, J., Boiron, M., Jacquillat, C., Weil, M., Levy, D., and Bernard, J.: Effects of rubidomycin in chronic myeloid leukemia. Path. Biol., 15:943, 1967.
8. Haut, A., Abbot, W. S., Wintrobe, M. M., and Cartwright, G. E.: Busulfan in the treatment of chronic myelocytic leukemia. The effect of long term intermittent therapy. Blood, 17:1–19, 1961.
9. Comparison of 6-mercaptopurine and busulfan in chronic granulocytic leukemia. Southeastern Cancer Chemotherapy Cooperative Study Group. Blood, 21:89–101, 1963.
10. Krebs, C., and Bichel, J.: Results of roentgen treatment in chronic myelogenous leukemia. Acta Radiol., 28:697, 1947.
11. Reinhard, E. H., Neely, L., and Samples, D. M.: Radioactive phosphorus in the treatment of chronic leukemias: Long-term results over a period of 15 years. Ann. Intern. Med., 50:942–958, 1959.
12. Karanas, A., and Silver, R. T.: Characteristics of the terminal phase of chronic granulocytic leukemia. Blood, 32:445–459, 1968.
13. Zubrod, C. G.: New developments in the chemotherapy of the leukemias and lymphomas. In Jaffe, E. (Editor): Plenary Session Papers, XII Congress, International Society of Hematology. New York, The Society, 1968, p. 32.
14. Green, R. A., and Dixon, H.: Expectancy for life in chronic lymphatic leukemia. Blood, 25:23–30, 1965.
15. Boggs, D. R., Sofferman, S. A., Wintrobe, M. M., and Cartwright, G. E.: Factors influencing the duration of survival of patients with chronic lymphocytic leukemia. Amer. J. Med., 40:243–254, 1966.
16. Rosenberg, S. A., Diamond, H. D., Jaslowitz, B., and Craver, L. F.: Lymphosarcoma: Review of 1,269 cases. Medicine, 40:31–84, 1961.
17. Horwitz, M. S., and Moore, G. T.: Acute infectious lymphocytosis. An etiologic and epidemiologic study of an outbreak. New Eng. J. Med., 279:399–404, 1968.
18. Putnam, S. M., Moore, G. T., and Mitchell, D. W.: Infectious lymphocytosis: Long-term follow-up of an epidemic. Pediatrics, 41:588, 1968.
19. Casey, T. P.: Chronic lymphocytic leukaemia in a child presenting at the age of two years and eight months. Australasian Ann. Med., 17:70–74, 1968.
20. Chervenick, P. A., Boggs, D. B., and Wintrobe, M. M.: Spontaneous remission in chronic lymphocytic leukemia. Ann. Intern. Med., 67:1239–1242, 1967.
21. Huguley, C. M.: Long-term study of chronic lymphocytic leukemia: Interim report after 45 months. Cancer Chemother. Rep., 16:241, 1962.
22. Ezdinli, E. Z., and Stutzman, L.: Chlorambucil therapy for lymphomas and chronic lymphocytic leukemia. J.A.M.A., 191:444–450, 1965.
23. Shaw, R. K., Boggs, D. R., Silberman, H. R., and Frei, E., III: A study of prednisone therapy in chronic lymphocytic leukemia. Blood, 17:182–195, 1961.
24. Johnson, R. E., Kagan, A. R., Gralnick, H. R., and Fass, L.: Radiation-induced remissions in chronic lymphocytic leukemia. Cancer, 20:1382–1387, 1967.
25. Osgood, E. E.: Treatment of chronic leukemia. J. Nuc. Med., 5:139–153, 1964.
26. Schrek, R.: Prednisolone sensitivity and cytology of viable lymphocytes as tests for chronic lymphocytic leukemia. J. Nat. Cancer Inst., 33:837–848, 1964.
27. Gardner, F. H., and Pringle, J. C.: Androgens and erythropoiesis. I. Preliminary clinical observations. Arch. Intern. Med., 107:846–862, 1961.
28. Rubin, A. D., Havemann, K., and Dameshek, W.: Studies in chronic lymphocytic

leukemia: Further studies of the proliferative abnormality of the blood lympho-cyte. Blood, *33*:313, 1969.

29. Cone, L., and Uhr, J. W.: Immunological deficiency disorders associated with chronic lymphocytic leukemia and multiple myeloma. J. Clin. Invest., *43*:2241–2248, 1964.

30. Miller, D. G., and Karnofsky, D. A.: Immunologic factors and resistance to infection in chronic lymphatic leukemia. Amer. J. Med., *31*:748–757, 1961.

31. Ultmann, J. E.: Generalized vaccinia in a patient with chronic lymphocytic leu-kemia and hypogammaglobulinemia. Ann. Intern. Med., *61*:728–732, 1964.

32. Cronkite, E. P.: Extracorporeal irradiation of the blood and lymph in the treatment of leukemia and for immunosuppression. Ann. Intern. Med., *67*:415, 1967.

33. Laszlo, J., Buckley, C. E., III, and Amos, D. B.: Infusion of isologous immune plasma in chronic lymphocytic leukemia. Blood, *31*:104–110, 1968.

Recent Additional Bibliography Not Cited in Text

34. Ezdinli, E. Z., Sokal, J. E., Crosswhite, L., and Sandberg, A. A.: Philadelphia-chromosome-positive and -negative chronic myelocytic leukemia. Ann. Intern. Med., *72*:175–182, 1970.

35. Tobin, M. S., Kyung-Suk-Kim, and Kossowsky, W. A.: Adrenocorticotrophic-hormone deficiency in chronic myelogenous leukemia after treatment. New Eng. J. Med., *282*:187, 1970.

CHAPTER 12

HODGKIN'S DISEASE AND OTHER LYMPHOMAS

A variety of classifications of the malignant lymphomas may be found in the literature. In Table 12-1, five major classes of lymphoma are listed.

Lymphoma may present either as an asymptomatic enlargement of a group of lymph nodes or as symptomatic disease characterized by fever, pallor, malaise, and weight loss. Hodgkin's disease is more often associated with fever and pruritus than are the other types of lymphoma. Reticulum cell sarcoma tends to be the most aggressive of these malignancies, and giant follicular lymphoma the most indolent. There are, however, numerous exceptions to this generalization. Reticulum cell sarcoma and lymphosarcoma arise in extralymphatic sites such as the gastrointestinal tract and nasopharynx in about one-third of the patients, whereas an extralymphatic origin is quite rare in Hodgkin's disease. Detailed descriptions of the clinical patterns and natural history of the lymphomas are available in standard textbooks of hematology.[1]

The diagnosis of lymphoma must be established by lymph node biopsy. The report of the pathologist will generally specify one of the types of lymphoma listed in Table 12-1. It may, in addition, further subdivide Hodgkin's disease into one of several histologic subtypes.

TABLE 12-1   *Classification of the Lymphomas*

Hodgkin's disease
Lymphosarcoma (also called small-cell lymphosarcoma)
Reticulum cell sarcoma (also called large-cell lymphosarcoma or lymphoblastic lymphosarcoma)
Giant follicular lymphosarcoma
Mycosis fungoides

CORRELATION OF HISTOLOGIC CLASSIFICATION, MODE OF SPREAD, AND PROGNOSIS

A new histologic classification of Hodgkin's disease,[2-4] supplanting the time-honored classification of Jackson and Parker,[5] has been found to be effective in predicting prognosis (see Table 12-2).[3] Nodular sclerosis is the largest histologic subgroup of Hodgkin's disease and has a favorable prognosis. The lymphocytic depletion subgroup has the least favorable prognosis. Prognosis also has a positive correlation with the apparent mode of spread of disease. The usual mode of spread of Hodgkin's disease of the nodular sclerosis variety is to adjacent lymph node groups in an orderly manner. Noncontiguous dissemination, with "skipping" of lymph node groups, is much more common in the lymphocytic depletion and mixed cellularity categories.

New histopathologic classifications that can be correlated with the natural history of disease and the response to treatment have not been established for the malignant lymphomas other than Hodgkin's disease.

EVALUATION OF THE PATIENT AND STAGING

Two observations are critical to the clinical approach to Hodgkin's disease: (1) In many instances, the disease appears to progress in an orderly manner from one group of lymph nodes to another adjacent group. (2) In localized disease, a sterilizing x-ray dose to the tumor kills or injures all tumor cells, so that local recurrence is prevented. From these observations has come the most important

TABLE 12-2   Histologic Classification of Hodgkin's Disease°

Category	Comments
1. Lymphocytic predominance	Includes paragranuloma of Jackson and Parker type[5] and lymphocytic and histiocytic types, nodular and diffuse.
2. Nodular sclerosis	A subdivision of granuloma based on the presence of collagenous bands.
3. Mixed cellularity	A subdivision of granuloma; a variety of cell types, including Reed-Sternberg cells, eosinophils, plasma cells, lymphocytes, neutrophils, and histiocytes. Slight to moderate fibrosis.
4. Lymphocytic depletion	Includes sarcoma of Jackson and Parker type[5] and diffuse fibrosis and reticular types of Lukes and Butler.[2]

°Adapted from Lukes, R. J., et al.: Report of the nomenclature committee. Cancer Res., 26 (Part I):1311, 1966.

advance in the past decade in the management of Hodgkin's disease: *Many patients with early lesions and localized disease can be cured by intensive local radiation therapy.*

More than half the patients with Hodgkin's disease have localized disease at the time of diagnosis and are potentially curable. Localized disease at the time of diagnosis is much less common in the other malignant lymphomas,[6] and the majority of these patients are probably not curable by intensive radiation therapy as it is currently used. Despite this, an attempt should be made to identify those few patients with lymphoma other than Hodgkin's disease whose tumor is still localized.

Because of the potential curability of localized disease, the clinical evaluation and therapeutic management of the patient with Hodgkin's disease have changed radically. Unfortunately, this fact is not universally appreciated, and, as stated recently in the New York Times,[7] "The death rates from Hodgkin's disease could probably be cut sharply if more doctors and their patients knew what they should about this form of cancer."

Initial Evaluation

The initial evaluation of the patient with lymphoma involves staging the disease.[8-10] If the disease is not obviously widespread at the time of diagnosis, clinical evaluation includes the following: a thorough physical examination, complete blood count, serum electrophoresis, chest roentgenograms and radiologic bone survey, radioisotopic bone scan (if facilities are available), intravenous pyelogram, lymphangiography to delineate pelvic lymph nodes, bone marrow biopsy, liver function tests, and radioisotopic liver scan. If palpation is inadequate to define a group of lymph nodes as positive or negative for Hodgkin's disease, then open biopsy is necessary. To this formidable list of tests some treatment centers add inferior vena cavography and skin sensitization to dinitrochlorobenzene.[9] In obviously widespread disease, liver biopsy, lymphangiography, and vena cavography are usually not necessary. Normal pulmonary function must be established prior to lymphangiography; microembolization of the lungs with oil droplets results from the procedure and may be fatal in the patient with pulmonary disease.

Staging

The clinical stage classification can usually be made on the basis of these extensive clinical studies. A recently proposed international staging classification for Hodgkin's disease is based on anatomic extent of disease (see Table 12-3).[11] Each stage is further subdivided into A or B, depending on whether the patient is asymptomatic (A) or

TABLE 12–3   *International Staging Classification for*
Hodgkin's Disease * †

Stage I:	Disease limited to one anatomic region or two contiguous anatomic regions on the same side of the diaphragm.
Stage II:	Disease in more than two anatomic regions or in two noncontiguous regions on the same side of the diaphragm.
Stage III:	Disease on both sides of the diaphragm but not extending beyond the involved lymph nodes and the spleen, or Waldeyer's ring.
Stage IV:	Involvement of bone marrow, lung, pleura, bone, liver, skin, kidney, gastrointestinal tract, or any tissue or organ, in addition to lymphatic system.

*Adapted from Rosenberg, S. A.: Report of the committee on staging of Hodgkin's disease. Cancer Res., 26:1310, 1966.

†Each stage is further divided into *A* (patient asymptomatic) or *B* (patient symptomatic, e.g., fever, night sweats, generalized pruritis).

has symptoms of fever, night sweats, or generalized pruritus (*B*). In general, the prognosis for patients in the *B* category is less favorable.

It should be stressed that only approximately 10 per cent of the patients with Hodgkin's disease have stage IV disease at the time of diagnosis, whereas roughly 30 to 60 per cent of the patients with other types of malignant lymphoma have widely disseminated disease at the time of diagnosis.[6] It should be stressed also that in evaluating the patient, even the detailed laboratory procedures just listed are insufficient for accurate staging about 25 per cent of the time, and in some experimental centers exploratory laparotomies are performed. Although it is my practice to recommend laparotomy for the accurate staging of most patients with Hodgkin's disease, this procedure cannot yet be recommended as "standard" for all practitioners.

The staging of other lymphomas is similar to that of Hodgkin's disease. Lymphomas arising in extralymphatic sites are staged differently. A tumor limited to a single extralymphatic site is classified as stage I (for example, a primary lymphoma restricted to the stomach or nasopharynx). If the regional nodes draining the primary site are involved, then the disease is considered stage II. Mycosis fungoides is generally regarded as disseminated (stage IV) disease.

THERAPEUTIC APPROACH AS A FUNCTION OF THE STAGE OF DISEASE

Staging is critical to the choice of therapy for the patient with lymphoma. This relationship is outlined in Figure 12-1 for Hodgkin's disease. Until more information is available about the results of radical radiation therapy in apparently localized lymphoma other than Hodgkin's disease, the same therapeutic approach should be

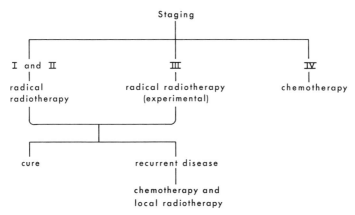

Figure 12-1   Therapeutic approach to Hodgkin's disease as a function of staging.

applied to other lymphomas (Fig. 12-1). Clearly, in stages I and II disease, radical supravoltage radiation therapy is indicated.[12-14] Technical details regarding such intensive radiation therapy are available in the literature.[15] The choice of therapy is less clear-cut in stage III disease. In my opinion, stage III patients should also be regarded as potentially curable by radical radiation therapy until more information is available to assess the long-term effectiveness of this mode of treatment. If radiation therapy fails to cure stage III disease, chemotherapy can subsequently be used.

When radiation is used with a curative intent, there is no place for simultaneous chemotherapy. Similarly, extirpative surgery has only one place in the treatment of lymphoma—in stage I disease, when the primary site is outside the lymphatic system.

CHEMOTHERAPY OF DISSEMINATED HODGKIN'S DISEASE

Chemotherapy is the standard treatment for patients with advanced (stage IV) disease. It may also be used to treat patients with recurrent stage III disease after radical therapy has failed.

The treatment of advanced Hodgkin's disease requires the sequential use of a number of drugs. The chemotherapy of other types of disseminated lymphoma involves a variation of the basic sequence of the agents used in Hodgkin's disease.

The agents and therapeutic programs available for the treatment of Hodgkin's disease may be categorized as standard (widely accepted) or experimental. The standard drugs are the commonly used alkylating agents (nitrogen mustard, chlorambucil, and cyclophosphamide), the vinca alkaloids (vinblastine and vincristine), procarbazine, and corticosteroids. Experimental agents and programs include

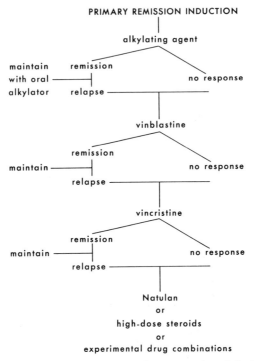

PRIMARY REMISSION INDUCTION

alkylating agent

maintain
with oral —————— remission
alkylator   no response

relapse ————————————

vinblastine

remission
maintain ——————   no response

relapse ————————————

vincristine

remission
maintain ——————   no response

relapse ————————————

Natulan
or
high-dose steroids
or
experimental drug combinations

Figure 12–2 Sequential treatment of disseminated Hodgkin's disease.

1,3-bis(β-chloroethyl)-1-nitrosourea (BCNU), colchicine analogues, cytosine arabinoside, and novel combinations of new and old agents.

The sequential treatment of advanced Hodgkin's disease is outlined in Figure 12-2. In most clinics, an alkylating agent is used for the initial treatment (primary induction of remission). The fact that an alkylating agent is usually the agent of choice reflects the effectiveness of these drugs and the extensive experience in using them. However, in one large published series, vinblastine was slightly superior to alkylators in the frequency of remission induction in previously untreated patients with Hodgkin's disease.[16] Vinblastine was not superior to alkylators in the primary treatment of other disseminated lymphomas.

Alkylating Agents

The dosage schedule for alkylating agents is given in Table 12-4. It appears likely that the commonly used alkylators are all equally effective if given in comparable doses.[17] If a rapid effect is desired, an alkylator that is effective intravenously is given; for slower induction, an orally effective agent suffices.

TABLE 12-4   *Dosage Schedules for Alkylating Agents (Hodgkin's Disease)*

Induction of remission
  Rapid — intravenous administration
    Nitrogen mustard: 0.4–0.5 mg./kg., divided doses
    Cyclophosphamide: 20–30 mg./kg., divided doses

  Slow — oral administration
    Cyclophosphamide: 2–3 mg./kg./day
    Chlorambucil: 0.05–0.1 mg./kg./day

Maintenance therapy — oral administration
  Cyclophosphamide: 2–3 mg./kg./day
  Chlorambucil: 0.05–0.1 mg./kg./day

Between 50 and 60 per cent of patients with previously untreated Hodgkin's disease can be expected to respond to such therapy. Most authorities agree that the duration of remission is prolonged with maintenance therapy.[16, 18] Low-dose oral maintenance treatment with cyclophosphamide is comparable in effectiveness to intermittent intensive therapy given intravenously (Table 12-4).

Vinblastine

Eventually the patient's disease relapses despite continued therapy. When the disease becomes "fast" to alkylators, vinblastine is used for re-induction. There appears to be no cross-resistance developed to alkylators and vinca alkaloids.[19] Vinblastine has been used according to the following schedule:[16] 0.1 mg. per kg. the first week; 0.2 mg. per kg. the second week; then 0.3 mg. per kg. weekly until the white blood count falls below 4000 per cu. mm., when the dose is decreased. The white blood count is maintained at or above 4000 per cu. mm. Smaller doses have been used with comparable results.[19] In one study, when vinblastine was given orally, the results compared favorably with those obtained with intravenous therapy;[20] however, oral therapy is not standard at the present time. Treatment with vinblastine is continued until the disease shows evidence of relapse.

Vincristine

The third drug to be used is vincristine. It is often effective at low doses so that undesirable side effects are rare and tend to be minimal. The main side effect of vincristine therapy is neuropathy (see Chap. 2); the compound has relatively little marrow depressive effect. For this reason vincristine may be used earlier in the course of disseminated Hodgkin's disease if the patient is suffering from the myelosuppressive effects of extensive x-ray therapy or drug therapy.

There is less statistical information available on the effectiveness of vincristine in Hodgkin's disease than is the case with alkylators or vinblastine. Vincristine has also been used in the treatment of lymphomas other than Hodgkin's disease.[16] There is no question, however, that this drug may be very effective in some patients with disseminated Hodgkin's disease. It is surprising that it shows so little overlap, in either side effects or development of resistance, with the closely related compound, vinblastine.

Vincristine should be started at small, weekly doses of 10 to 12 μg. per kg. given intravenously. If no response is seen in 2 to 3 weeks, the dose should be increased up to 25 μg. per kg. per week. Treatment should not be abandoned until the drug has been used for at least 6 to 8 weeks. If a remission has been induced by that time, it should be maintained with the minimal effective dose given weekly or every other week. A careful watch should be kept for the appearance of peripheral neuropathy, and stool softeners and cathartics should be used during treatment.

Natulan

Natulan (procarbazine, 1-methyl-2-p-(isopropyl-carbamoyl) benzylhydrazine) has been used with success in late stage Hodgkin's disease.[21] In adults, natulan is given initially in single or divided daily doses of 100 to 200 mg. for one week. If nausea and vomiting are not severe, the dosage is increased to 300 mg. daily and is maintained at that level until (1) the white blood count falls below 4000 per cu. mm. or the platelet count falls below 100,000 per cu. mm. or (2) a maximal antitumor response is achieved. If there is evidence of hematopoietic depression or central nervous system toxicity, administration of the drug is stopped until there has been a satisfactory recovery. A dosage schedule of 50 to 100 mg. daily is used once a remission has been achieved. Therapy is continued until evidence of drug resistance appears. Smaller than usual doses are used if renal or hepatic functional abnormalities are present.

In addition to hematopoietic depression, the principal side effects of natulan therapy include nausea, vomiting, and central nervous system toxicity (see Chap. 2).

Corticosteroids

Hall[22] has recently reviewed the literature and summarized his own experience with the high-dose corticosteroid treatment in Hodgkin's disease and other lymphomas. He used prednisone in doses of 45 to 300 mg. per day for 3 to 75 weeks; other steroids were used at comparable or higher doses (up to 600 mg. per day). Worthwhile objective responses occurred in 66 per cent of the patients with Hodgkin's disease. Side effects were said to be infrequent and controllable. It must be stressed, however, that in most studies of the use of high-dose corticosteroids in disease other than Hodgkin's disease, the incidence of serious complications has been significant. It has been our practice, therefore, to restrict the use of steroids to treating those patients who are clearly resistant to the other modes of therapy, or to the treatment of complicating hemolytic anemia[23] or severe thrombocytopenia resulting from increased platelet destruction.

Recent Developments

When the alkylating agents, vinca alkaloids, procarbazine, and corticosteroids can no longer be used, all subsequent therapy must be considered investigational. The role of investigational agents such as BCNU remains to be evaluated.[24, 25] Some of these new agents were discussed at a recent clinical staff conference at the National Cancer Institute[26] and in an address to the International Society of Hematology.[27]

An exciting recent development is the use of combination chemotherapy.[28] A recent report by DeVita and Serpick[29] describes truly startling results with combination therapy in far-advanced Hodgkin's disease. These studies, although preliminary, hold great promise for the future and clearly indicate that standard therapy may change radically within the next few years.

CHEMOTHERAPY OF OTHER MALIGNANT LYMPHOMAS

Although there are distinct differences in the natural history and response to therapy among the malignant lymphomas,[30] the general therapeutic program outlined for disseminated Hodgkin's disease is applicable to other disseminated lymphomas.

Giant follicular lymphosarcoma tends to be a relatively indolent disease in at least half the patients; near the end of its course it may be transformed into a disease closely resembling reticulum cell sarcoma.[31] During its indolent phase it is usually best treated by local radiation therapy alone. Reticulum cell sarcoma tends to be the most aggressive of the lymphomas and is usually the least responsive to chemotherapy. As a general rule, lymphosarcoma occupies a place intermediate between giant follicular lymphosarcoma and reticulum cell sarcoma in terms of virulence. Like all general rules, there are many exceptions. Both lymphosarcoma and reticulum cell sarcoma may involve the bone marrow and peripheral blood and produce a clinical picture somewhere in the spectrum between acute lymphocytic and chronic lymphocytic leukemia. When this occurs, therapy appropriate to acute lymphocytic leukemia should probably be used.

Alkylating agents are the drugs of choice in the primary treatment of disseminated lymphomas. Cyclophosphamide may be effective in producing worthwhile responses in 40 to 70 per cent of the patients with reticulum cell sarcoma and lymphosarcoma.[16, 32] The drug should be continued at a maintenance dosage after induction of remission. It is doubtful, however, that such remissions significantly prolong the life of the patient with reticulum cell sarcoma.[32, 33] When disease becomes resistant to alkylating agents, vincristine should be used; between 17 and 40 per cent of previously treated patients can expect to benefit from vincristine.[16] Vinblastine can be tried subsequently, although there are fewer data available to assess its effectiveness. Thereafter, all chemotherapy must be regarded as investigational.

Mycosis fungoides is an interesting lymphoma with a unique natural history and histogenesis.[34] Many modalities of therapy have been used, including irradiation with x-rays or with high-energy electrons; systemic therapy with alkylating agents, methotrexate, and corticosteroids; topical application of nitrogen mustard; and topical application of 2,4-dinitrochlorobenzene to previously sensitized subjects. All have been reported to produce beneficial effects in small groups of patients. Recently Waldorf et al.[35] have documented some of the cellular changes that occur with several types of therapy.

In the patient whose disease is largely confined to the skin, one form of treatment at present consists of electron-beam irradiation and local "spotting" of thickened plaques with orthovoltage x-rays. When the disease is no longer controllable by ionizing irradiation or when it is extensive and involves the viscera, systemic chemotherapy should be used.[35, 36]

Cyclophosphamide was introduced in the treatment of mycosis fungoides by Abele and Dobson[37] in 1960. It is probably the first agent of choice for the control of systemic disease. A recent report suggests that chlorpromazine may be useful in combination with cyclophosphamide.[38] This remains to be confirmed by a more extensive study.

Patients whose disease becomes resistant to alkylating agents should be given trials with other agents, as shown in Figure 12-2, the sequential scheme of chemotherapy recommended for advanced Hodgkin's disease.

Topical nitrogen mustard has been tried in the treatment of mycosis fungoides.[39] Insufficient data have accumulated to assess its value. My own experience with this form of treatment has been limited and the patients have had severe toxic reactions.

The direct imposition of delayed hypersensitivity reactions to dinitrochlorobenzene on mycosis fungoides lesions is new and inno-vative.[40] It is unlikely to be a generally useful therapeutic tool.

TREATMENT OF COMPLICATIONS

It is important to emphasize that the complications and clinical problems associated with malignant lymphomas are often best treated by local radiation therapy. Thus, disfiguring accumulations of enlarged lymph nodes, superior vena cava obstruction, and ureteral blockage often respond best to appropriate x-ray therapy. The clinical problems frequently associated with malignant lymphoma are outlined in Table 12-5, as are the appropriate therapeutic approaches.

Spinal Cord Compression

Spinal cord compression from an extradural lymphomatous mass is a problem frequently encountered on an oncology service. One point is clear: *The appearance of symptoms of compression always constitutes a medical emergency.*[41, 42] Treatment should be prompt, and requires the combined efforts of the neurosurgeon, the radiation therapist, and the chemotherapist. (See Chapter 14 on the treatment of complications.)

ILLUSTRATIVE CASE HISTORY: HODGKIN'S DISEASE

A student was first seen at the University of California Hospitals, San Francisco, in 1966, when he was 16 years old. One year previously he had

TABLE 12-5   *Treatment of Associated Problems in Malignant Lymphoma*

SYMPTOM	MODE OF TREATMENT
Fever	Aspirin (often poor response)
	Aminopyrine (in addition to primary therapy)
Superior vena cava syndrome	Radiation therapy and chemotherapy
Pleural effusions	Drainage of fluid
	Nitrogen mustard or Thiotepa, intrapleurally
	Atabrine (rarely)
Pericardial effusions	Drainage of fluid
	Radiation therapy
	Pericardiectomy (rarely)
Genitourinary obstruction	Radiation therapy and chemotherapy
Infection	Antibiotics
Hemolytic anemia	Corticosteroids
"Hypersplenism"	Corticosteroids as primary therapy
	Splenectomy in selected patients
Hyperuricemia	Allopurinol

noticed a painless swelling in the left axilla, and then additional masses appeared in the left supraclavicular fossa and right axilla. He had no fever, weight loss, or pruritis, and did not seek medical attention until two weeks before hospital admission in *May 1966*. At that time a biopsy of the left axillary lymph node established a diagnosis of Hodgkin's disease.

The findings of the physical examination were within normal limits, except for lymphadenopathy in the areas described. The results of the following laboratory studies were within normal limits: bone marrow biopsy, complete blood count, liver function, intravenous pyelogram, radioisotopic survey of bones, radioisotopic liver scan, and inferior vena cavagram. Abdominal lymphangiography was performed after a determination of normal pulmonary diffusion capacity. Roentgenograms of the chest showed a right paratracheal mass. The patient's disease was classified as stage IIA, and radiation therapy with curative intent was begun to the cervical, mediastinal, and axillary lymph node-bearing areas. (A subsequent course of abdominal irradiation had been planned.)

In *November 1966*, four months after completion of a course of radiation therapy (4500 rads in a mantle distribution), the patient complained of low back pain and fever. An abdominal mass was felt. A repeat lymphangiogram revealed involvement of the inguinal and periaortic lymph nodes (Fig. 12–3). The findings of bone marrow biopsy were considered to be consistent with infiltration by Hodgkin's disease (fibrotic nodules with reticulum cells but no Reed-Sternberg cells). The disease was therefore reclassified as stage IVB.

Because the patient was symptomatic and had stage IV disease, chemotherapy was begun immediately. The dose of nitrogen mustard was small (0.25 mg. per kg.) because of previous radiation therapy and bone marrow involvement. One month later the patient felt well and was free of symptoms. The white blood count and the platelet count were normal and the abdominal mass was no longer palpable. The nodes seen on the lymphangiogram to contain the radiopaque dye had shrunk (Fig. 12–4).

Maintenance therapy with chlorambucil was begun. The patient continued to look and feel well for 10 months. After this asymptomatic interval, back pain developed; an osteoblastic lesion of the tenth thoracic vertebra was found. No other evidence of active disease was noted, and local radiation therapy was given to the spinal area involved. Chlorambucil administration was continued.

Three months after completing radiation therapy (*January 1968*), the patient was anemic and the cervical masses had recurred; he complained of weakness and night sweats. When the patient was re-evaluated, exacerbation of disease was evident. Recurrent involvement of the external and common iliac nodes was found. Treatment with vinblastine was begun, 0.1 mg. per kg. per week. Within 2 weeks an impressive regression of all abnormal nodes was noted.

Remission of disease was sustained for approximately 10 months with doses of vinblastine averaging 0.15 mg. per kg. given weekly or every other week. In *October 1968*, when cervical lymphadenopathy recurred, vinblastine was stopped and vincristine was started. The dose was 1 mg. given weekly or every other week; a careful watch was kept for the appearance of neuropathy.

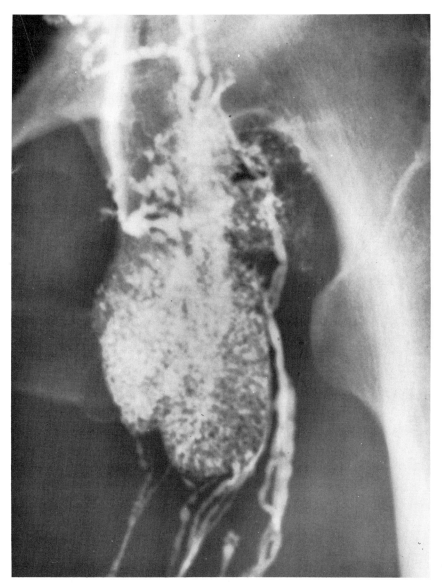

Figure 12-3 Lymphangiogram of a patient with Hodgkin's disease, showing a lymph node invaded by tumor. See case history.

After a period of 10 weeks during which the disease was in good control, lymphadenopathy and systemic symptoms reappeared. At this time the patient's disease was considered to be resistant to both alkylating agents and vinca alkaloids. Consequently, therapy was Natulan (procarbazine) was initiated according to an experimental protocol in which the dose was 200 mg. per day for 14 days and thereafter 25 to 50 mg. per day. Despite the development of neutropenia, a good response to therapy was evident within

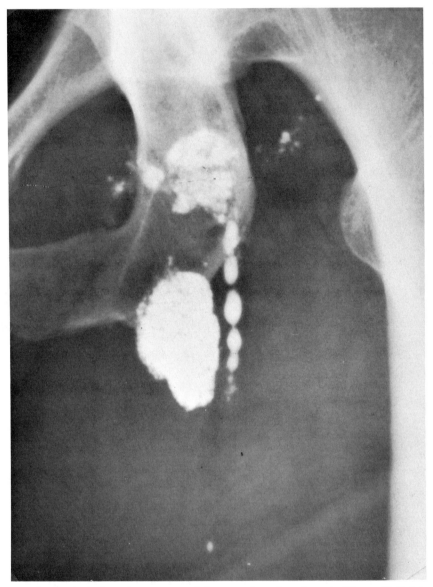

Figure 12–4 Lymphangiogram of the same lymph node as in Figure 12–3, following chemotherapy.

2 weeks, and the disease was in remission after 4 weeks. Natulan therapy was effective for 2 months; during this period the patient felt entirely well.

The patient was hospitalized again late in *March 1969* with pleural effusions, pulmonary infiltrates, and enlarging inguinal lymph nodes (Fig. 12-5). A pleural biopsy was consistent with Hodgkin's disease.

Natulan therapy was discontinued and experimental therapy with BCNU was begun. Within 10 days the pulmonary infiltrate had disappeared and all palpable lymph nodes had shrunk to normal size (Fig. 12–6). One month later, however, he returned to the hospital with pancytopenia and fever. An infectious etiology for the fever could not be ascertained.

Treatment with BCNU was discontinued and prednisone, 30 mg. per day, was begun. The fever disappeared and the patient felt well for about 6 weeks. He then returned to the hospital because of enlarging nodes and recurrent pleural effusions. Intensive chemotherapy was precluded by pancytopenia. On *July 1, 1969*, the patient died of pneumonia and uncontrolled bleeding, 4 years after his initial symptoms had appeared.

COMMENT: When this patient's disease was found to be disseminated to an extent presently considered to be incurable by radiation

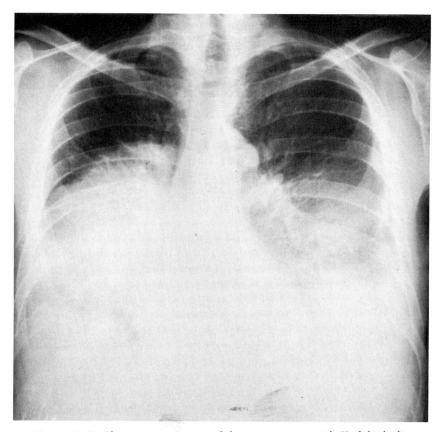

Figure 12–5 Chest roentgenogram of the same patient with Hodgkin's disease as in Figure 12–3, showing pulmonary infiltration.

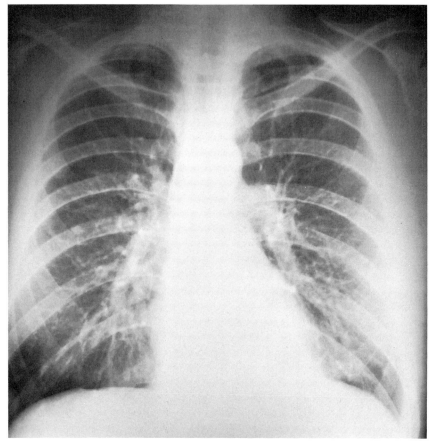

Figure 12-6 Chest roentgenogram of the same patient as in Figure 12–3, after therapy with BCNU (1,3-bis(β-chloroethyl)-1-nitrosourea).

therapy, sequential chemotherapy with standard agents (alkylators, vinblastine, vincristine, Natulan) induced and maintained a series of remissions extending over a period of 28 months. Thereafter, experimental drugs and prednisone were used for the subsequent three months of life. (See Figure 12–2.)

REFERENCES

1. Wintrobe, M. M.: *Clinical Hematology.* Ed. 6. Philadelphia, Lea & Febiger, 1967, Chapter 20.
2. Lukes, R. J., and Butler, J. J.: The pathology and nomenclature of Hodgkin's disease. Cancer Res., 26:1063, 1966.
3. Keller, A. R., Kaplan, H. S., Lukes, R. J., and Rappaport, H.: Correlation of histopathology with other prognostic indicators in Hodgkin's disease. Cancer, 22:487, 1968.
4. Lukes, R. J., Craver, L. F., Hall, T. C., Rappaport, H., and Ruben, P.: Report of the

nomenclature committee. *In* Symposium: Obstacles to the control of Hodgkin's disease. Cancer Res., *26*(Part I):1311, 1966

5. Jackson, H., Jr., and Parker, F., Jr.: Hodgkin's disease. II. Pathology. New Eng. J. Med., *231*:35, 1944.

6. Kaplan, H. S., and Rosenberg, S. A: Cure of Hodgkin's disease and other malignant lymphomas. Postgrad. Med., *43*:146, 1968.

7. The New York Times, February 3, 1967.

8. Karnofsky, D. A.: The staging of Hodgkin's disease. Cancer Res., *26*:1090, 1966.

9. Brown, R. S., Haynes, H. A., Foley, H. T., Godwin, H. A., Berard, C. W., and Carbone, P. P.: Hodgkin's disease. Immunologic, clinical, and histologic features of 50 untreated patients. Ann. Intern. Med., *67*:291–302, 1967.

10. Gellhorn, A.: A new look at lymphomas. Postgrad. Med., *43*:136, 1968.

11. Rosenberg, S. A.: Report of the committee on staging of Hodgkin's disease. Cancer Res., *26*:1310, 1966.

12. Peters, M. V.: Prophylactic treatment of adjacent areas in Hodgkin's disease. Cancer Res., *26*:1232–1243, 1966.

13. Easson, E. C.: Long-term results of radical radiotherapy in Hodgkin's disease. Cancer Res., *26*:1244–1249, 1966.

14. Kaplan, H. S.: Long-term results of palliative and radical radiotherapy of Hodgkin's disease. Cancer Res., *26*:1250–1253, 1966.

15. Kaplan, H. S.: Role of intensive radiotherapy in the management of Hodgkin's disease. Cancer, *19*:356, 1966.

16. Carbone, P. P., and Spurr, C.: Management of patients with malignant lymphoma: A comparative study with cyclophosphamide and vinca alkaloids. Cancer Res., *28*:811, 1968.

17. Jacobs, E. M., Peters, F. C., Luce, J. K., Zippin, C., and Wood, D. A.: Mechlorethamine HCl and cyclophosphamide in the treatment of Hodgkin's disease and the lymphomas. J.A.M.A., *203*:392–398, 1968.

18. Scott, J. L.: The effect of nitrogen mustard and chlorambucil in the treatment of advanced Hodgkin's disease. Cancer Chemother. Rep., *27*:27–32, 1963.

19. Sohier, W. D., Wong, R. K. L., and Aisenberg, A. C.: Vinblastine in the treatment of advanced Hodgkin's disease. Cancer, *22*:467, 1968.

20. Wilson, H. E., and Louis, J.: The response of Hodgkin's disease to treatment with oral vinblastine sulfate. Ann. Intern. Med., *67*:303, 1967.

21. Hansen, M. M., Hertz, H., and Videbaek, A.: Use of a methyl hydrazine derivative (Natulan), especially in Hodgkin's disease. Acta Med. Scand., *180*(Fasc. 2):211–224, 1966.

22. Hall, T. C., Choi, O. S., Abadi, A., and Krant, M. J.: High-dose corticosteroid therapy in Hodgkin's disease and other lymphomas. Ann. Intern. Med., *66*:1144, 1967.

23. Cline, M. J., and Berlin, N. L.: Anemia in Hodgkin's disease. Cancer, *16*:526, 1963.

24. Lessner, H. E.: BCNU (1,3 bis-(β-chloroethyl)-1-nitrosourea). Cancer, *22*:451, 1968.

25. Carter, S. K., and Newman, J. W.: Nitrosoureas. Cancer Chemother. Rep., *1*:115, 1968.

26. Clinical Staff Conference, National Cancer Institute: Hodgkin's disease. Ann. Intern. Med., *67*:424, 1967.

27. Zubrod, C. G.: New developments in the chemotherapy of the leukemias and lymphomas. *In* Plenary Session Papers, XII Congress, International Society of Hematology. New York, 1968, p. 32.

28. Moxley, J. H., III, DeVita, V. T., Brace, K., and Frei, E., III: Intensive combination chemotherapy and X-irradiation in Hodgkin's disease. Cancer Res., *27*:1258–1263, 1967.

29. DeVita, V. T., and Serpick, A.: Combination chemotherapy in the treatment of advanced Hodgkin's disease. Proc. Amer. Assoc. Cancer Res., *8*:13, 1967.

30. Rosenberg, S. A., Diamond, H. D., Jaslowitz, B., and Craver, L. F.: Lymphosarcoma: A review of 1269 cases. Medicine, *40*:31, 1961.

31. Firat, D., Stutzman, L., Studensky, E. R., and Pickren, J.: Giant follicular lymph node disease. Clinical and pathological review of 64 cases. Amer. J. Med., *39*:252, 1965.

32. Hyman, G. A., and Cassileth, P. A.: Efficacy of cyclophosphamide in the management of reticulum cell sarcoma. Cancer, *19*:1386, 1966.

33. Gellhorn, A.: End-results in lymphosarcoma and Hodgkin's disease. *In* Proceed-

ings of the Third National Cancer Conference. Philadelphia, J. B. Lippincott Co., 1957, p. 862.

34. Block, J. B., Edgcomb, J., Eisen, A., and Van Scott, E. J.: Mycosis fungoides. Natural history and aspects of its relationship to other malignant lymphomas. Amer. J. Med., 34:228–235, 1963.

35. Waldorf, D. S., Ratner, A. C., and Van Scott, E. J.: Cells in lesions of mycosis fungoides lymphoma following therapy. Cancer, 21:264–269, 1967.

36. Clinicopathologic Conference. Mycosis fungoides with pulmonary and neurologic complications. Amer. J. Med., 42:129, 1967.

37. Abele, D. C., and Dobson, R. L.: The treatment of mycosis fungoides with a new agent, cyclophosphamide (Cytoxan). Arch. Derm., 82:725, 1960.

38. Maguire, A.: Treatment of mycosis fungoides with cyclophosphamide and chlorpromazine. Brit. J. Derm., 80:54, 1968.

39. Madison, J. F., and Haserick, J. R.: Topically applied mechlorethamine on 12 dermatoses. Arch. Derm., 86:663, 1962.

40. Ratner, A. E., Waldorf, D. S., and Van Scott, E. J.: Alteration of mycosis fungoides lymphoma by direct imposition of delayed hypersensitivity reactions. Cancer, 21:83, 1968.

41. Mones, R. J., Dozier, D., and Berrett, A.: Analysis of medical treatment of malignant extradural spinal cord tumors. Cancer, 19:1842, 1966.

42. Diamond, H. D., Williams, H. M., and Craver, L. F.: The pathogenesis and management of neurological complications of malignant lymphomas and leukemia. Cancer, 16:831, 1960.

Additional Recent Bibliography Not Cited in Text

43. Rapoport, A., Cole, P., and Mason, J.: Correlates of survival after initiation of chemotherapy in 142 cases of Hodgkin's disease. Cancer, 24:377–381, 1969.

44. Lowenbraun, S., Ramsey, H., Sutherland, J., and Serpick, A. A.: Diagnostic laparotomy and splenectomy for staging Hodgkin's disease. Ann. Intern. Med., 72:655–663, 1970.

45. Curran, R. E., and Johnson, R. E.: Tolerance to chemotherapy after prior irradiation for Hodgkin's disease. Ann. Intern. Med., 72:505–509, 1970.

46. Hoogstraten, B., Owens, A. H., Lenhard, R. E., Glidewell, O. J., Leone, L. A., Olson, K. B., Harley, J. B., Townsend, S. R., Miller, S. P., and Spurr, C. L.: Combination chemotherapy in lymphosarcoma and reticulum cell sarcoma. Blood, 33:370–378, 1969.

47. Lowenbraun, S., DeVita, V. T., and Serpick, A. A.: Combination chemotherapy with nitrogen mustard, vincristine, procarbazine, and prednisone in lymphosarcoma and reticulum cell sarcoma. Cancer, 25:1018–1025, 1970.

CHAPTER 13

MULTIPLE MYELOMA AND MACROGLOBULINEMIA

MULTIPLE MYELOMA

Several excellent recent reviews of the natural history and biology of multiple myeloma are available.[1-3] The malignant proliferation of plasma cells is expressed in a variety of clinical syndromes, which range from an asymptomatic increase in a homogeneous serum gamma globulin to a fulminant disease characterized by bony destruction, hematologic abnormalities, and often renal failure. The major clinical manifestations are summarized in Table 13–1. *In multiple myeloma one treats both the neoplastic proliferation of plasma cells and the secondary manifestations of this proliferation* (for example, hypercalcemia, hyperviscosity, and infection). In this disorder, supportive therapy is a critical adjunct to successful chemotherapy.

TABLE 13–1   *Clinical Manifestations of Multiple Myeloma*

Common
> Hypercalcemia
> Plasmacytosis of the bone marrow
> Homogeneous "spike" in the serum gamma globulins
> Bence Jones proteinuria, renal failure, or both
> Lytic bone lesions or osteoporosis
> Anemia
> Leukopenia
> Infection

Infrequent or rare
> Hyperviscosity syndrome, with visual disturbances, coma, others
> Spinal cord compression
> Amyloidosis

Specific Therapy

In the malignant plasma cell disorders, as in other malignant diseases, it is important to have objective criteria of the response to therapy. The relief of pain and an increase in the patient's activity, although difficult to quantitate, are most important. Objective criteria include decreases in serum myeloma protein concentration and urinary Bence Jones protein; control of anemia, renal insufficiency, and hypercalcemia; and reduction of bone marrow plasmacytosis. Although arrest of lytic bone lesions often occurs with chemotherapy, recalcification is rare.[4] It is likely, but not proved, that in man the serum concentration of myeloma protein reflects the size of the plasma cell mass.[5]

Among the cytotoxic drugs, only alkylating agents have been consistently useful in the treatment of the malignant plasma cell disorders. Melphalan, a phenylalanine derivative of nitrogen mustard, and cyclophosphamide have been most widely used and can be expected to produce an objective beneficial response in approximately 30 per cent of the patients with multiple myeloma.

MELPHALAN. Melphalan is available in 2 mg. tablets. Continuous daily therapy,[6] initial loading doses followed by smaller maintenance levels,[7] and intermittent intensive courses[8] have all been used. In general, the level of the white blood count has been used as the guide to treatment and is usually maintained in the range, 3000 to 4000 per cu. mm.; the white blood count should not be permitted to fall below 2000 per cu. mm. In occasional patients, thrombocytopenia rather than leukopenia is the dose-limiting sign of toxicity and may necessitate discontinuing the treatment.

In a cooperative study (cited in reference 2), a comparison was made of the effectiveness of melphalan given intermittently in high dosages (0.25 mg. per kg. per day on 4 successive days, repeated at 6-week intervals) and daily administration of 0.025 mg. per kg. The high-dosage schedule was found to be more effective.[2] This intermittent dosage schedule is the one currently recommended here. Somewhat larger daily maintenance doses (0.05 mg. per kg.), given to the point of leukopenia and then reduced in amount, may be effective in producing prolonged remissions.[6] Such treatment should be continued for at least 12 weeks.

The dosage schedules of melphalan and cyclophosphamide in multiple myeloma and chlorambucil in macroglobulinemia are outlined in Table 13-2. It is clear that the patients whose disease responds to alkylating agents live longer than nonresponders.[1, 4]

CYCLOPHOSPHAMIDE. Cyclophosphamide is about as effective as melphalan in inducing a remission and prolonging life in patients with multiple myeloma. It can be expected to induce remissions in 30 to 50 per cent of the patients.[9] Cyclophosphamide is given in

TABLE 13–2 *Dosage Schedules for Multiple*
Myeloma and Macroglobulinemia

DRUG	DOSAGE SCHEDULE (ORAL)	REFERENCE
Multiple myeloma		
Melphalan	1. 0.25 mg./kg./day x 4; repeated at 4- to 6-week intervals	2, 4
	2. 0.05 mg./kg./day until WBC falls below 5000/cu. mm.; then adjusted to maintain WBC between 2000 and 4000/cu. mm.	6
Cyclophosphamide	1–3 mg./kg./day; adjusted to maintain WBC between 2000 and 4000/cu. mm.	6
Macroglobulinemia		
Chlorambucil	0.025–0.1 mg./kg./day; adjusted to maintain WBC between 2000 and 4000/cu. mm.	18

dosages of 1 to 3 mg. per kg. per day until the white blood count falls below 4000 to 5000 per cu. mm. Thereafter, the dosage is adjusted downward to keep the white count above 2000 and preferably between 3000 and 4000 per cu. mm. In addition to myelosuppression, the complications of cyclophosphamide treatment include alopecia and hemorrhagic cystitis.

Melphalan and cyclophosphamide have been reported to produce beneficial results in some of the unusual variants of multiple myeloma, including extraosseous tumors,[10] acute renal failure,[11] and plasmacytic leukemia.[12]

Adrenocorticosteroids are used in the treatment of hypercalcemic complications of multiple myeloma (see following section, "Supportive Therapy"). Their use in the primary treatment of this disorder is not established, although they have benefited some patients.[6]

A preliminary report indicates that sodium fluoride may increase bone density in some patients with multiple myeloma.[13] The general efficacy of this agent, however, has still not been established. In my experience, gastrointestinal intolerance is the major problem associated with long-term sodium fluoride therapy.

A question frequently asked by the physician is when chemotherapy should be started in treating the patient with multiple myeloma. Most authorities agree that treatment should be started when the diagnosis is established. The disease is almost always inexorably progressive, and spontaneous remission or regression is virtually unknown. *Treatment should be started early.*

Supportive Therapy

HYPERCALCEMIA.   Hypercalcemia is a frequent manifestation of multiple myeloma, which, if uncontrolled, leads to gastrointestinal and neurologic disturbances, renal failure, and ultimately death. Often hypercalcemia can be controlled by adequate hydration, ambulation, and diminished calcium intake. Usually, however, adrenocorticosteroids (for example, prednisone, 60 to 80 mg. per day) are required to control severe hypercalcemia. They appear to work by reducing calcium resorption from bone.[14] Occasionally steroids fail and oral phosphate solutions may be required.[15] Phosphates, however, are not without their own hazards and must be used with caution. The intravenous use of phosphates is extremely hazardous and is not recommended.

RENAL FAILURE.   In general, this complication of myeloma responds poorly to either supportive therapy or specific chemotherapy. In occasional patients, however, gratifying results can be achieved by high fluid intake, treatment of complicating renal infection, and specific chemotherapy.

LYTIC BONE LESIONS.   Symptomatic bone lesions, such as collapsed vertebrae, are usually best treated by local radiation therapy. Although recalcification is infrequently achieved, symptomatic relief is often possible. Spinal cord compression is treated by radiotherapeutic and neurosurgical decompression, and sometimes chemotherapy. (See Chap. 14.) Supportive bracing of an involved spine is often necessary for ambulation.

ANEMIA.   The complex anemia of multiple myeloma[16] is best treated by androgens such as fluoxymesterone, 40 mg. per day, or depotestosterone, 600 to 1200 mg. per week. Some patients cannot tolerate such therapy because of virilization, fluid retention, or change in personality. Fluoxymesterone may produce cholestatic jaundice.

INFECTION.   Bacterial infections should be treated promptly with antibiotics after the appropriate cultures have been obtained and usually before the organisms have had time to grow out. *Because of the poor immune response of these patients, live vaccines such as vaccinia should be avoided.* Catastrophic complications result from casual vaccinations. The role of prophylactic gamma globulin or normal plasma in preventing infections in these patients is still uncertain.[17]

HYPERVISCOSITY SYNDROME.   This relatively rare complication of multiple myeloma is usually manifested by visual disturbances and occasionally neurologic disturbances accompanied by alteration of consciousness. If the problem is acute, vigorous plasmapheresis can be tried, although it is not usually as successful in reducing viscosity in multiple myeloma as in macroglobulinemia. In the slowly evolving clinical condition, specific antineoplastic chemotherapy is a more reliable method of reducing serum protein concentration and viscosity.

Recent Developments

An important new development, which probably will have implications for the management of many human malignancies, is a technique for the measurement of the total-body mass of myeloma tumor cells.[17a] The technique is based on measurements of the rate of synthesis of myeloma globulins by isolated plasma cells in vitro and of the size and turnover of the total-body pool of myeloma globulins in vivo. This technique puts the measurement of tumor cell mass in man on a firm experimental footing and obviates the necessity for theoretical extrapolations from animal tumor models (See Chap. 15.) Armed with such a method, one can determine the extremely long natural history of multiple myeloma (20 years or more) and document the very slow rate of replication of myeloma cells. In addition, one can precisely document the effects of therapy on the numbers and rate of replication of malignant cells. This technique provides a "marker," which may prove to be as precise and sensitive as the production of gonadotropic hormones by choriocarcinoma.

ILLUSTRATIVE CASE HISTORY: MULTIPLE MYELOMA

A 55-year-old man consulted his physician because of weakness and persistent low back pain following a fall. He was found to be anemic and to have proteinurea, and was referred to the University of California Hospitals, San Francisco, for evaluation in *February 1969*. He appeared pale and chronically ill. At physical examination there was tenderness to palpation over the lumbar spine. His hematocrit was 22 per cent, with 1.8 per cent reticulocyte count and a normal mean corpuscular hemoglobin concentration. The white blood count and platelet count were normal (Fig. 13-1). The total serum protein was 7.1 gm. per 100 ml. Electrophoresis of the serum showed a spike in the gamma globulin region (Fig. 13-2); this was subsequently characterized as an IgG kappa chain paraprotein. The serum calcium was 9.4 mg. per 100 ml. Myeloma cells comprised approximately 80 per cent of the bone marrow aspirate (Fig. 13-3). A bone survey showed generalized osteoporosis.

Treatment with melphalan was begun in 4-day courses of 0.25 mg. per kg. per day; each course was repeated at monthly intervals. The progress of his therapy is shown in Figures 13-1 and 13-2. The peripheral white blood count was maintained in the range of 4000 to 5000 per cu. mm. After 3 months of melphalan therapy a rise in the hematocrit was apparent; after 4 months there was a significant decrease in serum paraprotein concentration; by the sixth month of therapy no abnormal protein was apparent with serum electrophoresis (Fig. 13-2), although immunoelectrophoresis still revealed paraprotein. As judged by a radiologic survey, there had been no progression of bone disease over a 6-month period. The patient felt well and was active.

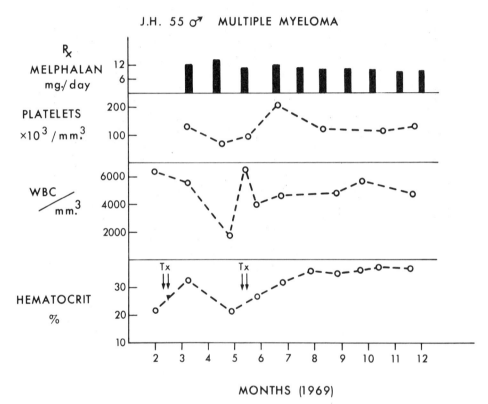

Figure 13–1 Response of a patient with multiple myeloma to therapy with melphalan. See case history.

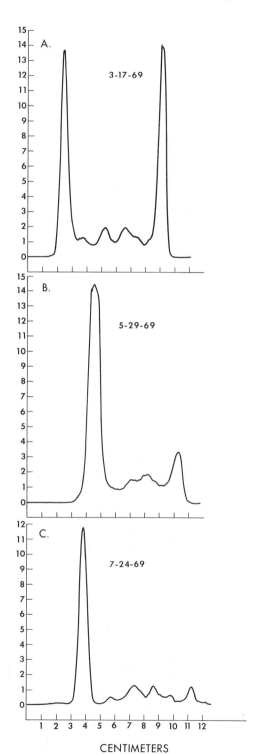

Figure 13–2 Serial electrophoresis of serum of the same patient with multiple myeloma showed gradual diminution of the myeloma protein "spike" during chemotherapy. See case history.

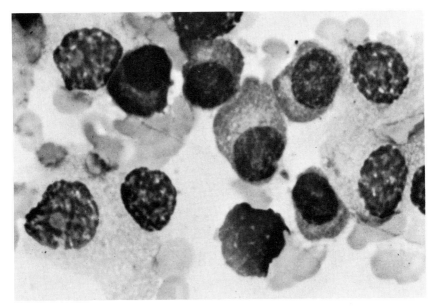

Figure 13–3   Bone marrow aspirate of the same patient with multiple myeloma before therapy with melphalan. (Original magnification, 1250 ×.)

COMMENT: The hematocrit and level of serum paraprotein were used as objective guides of this patient's response to melphalan therapy. The slow decrease in paraprotein concentration observed is typical of disease responsive to therapy. As is usual in multiple myeloma, there was no radiologic evidence of healing of the osteolytic lesions despite a response to therapy.

MACROGLOBULINEMIA

The clinical features and natural history of macroglobulinemia are considerably different from those of multiple myeloma.[2, 18, 19] Life expectancy is appreciably longer in macroglobulinemia than in multiple myeloma, and osteolytic lesions, hypercalcemia, renal failure, and amyloidosis are quite rare in macroglobulinemia. Susceptibility to infection is less common than in multiple myeloma. The hyperviscosity syndrome is, however, much more prominent in patients with macroglobulinemia than in those with myeloma, owing to the large size of the immunoglobulin and its restriction to the vascular space. The manifestations of the hyperviscosity syndrome include visual disturbance associated with retinal hemorrhage and a characteristic "sausage linking" of the retinal veins; occasional disturbances of consciousness and more profound central nervous system symptoms, sometimes progressing to coma; rare pulmonary hypertension; and right-sided congestive heart failure. The signs and symptoms of the hyperviscosity syndrome are often temporarily improved by intensive plasmapheresis.[20] For long-term control, however, chemotherapy is generally more reliable and certainly less trouble.

Chlorambucil has been the most extensively used chemotherapeutic agent and is generally successful[18] (see Table 13–2). Cyclophosphamide has also been used, but there is considerably less experience with this agent.[21] Anemia complicating macroglobulinemia may be treated with adrenocorticosteroids, androgens, or chlorambucil, depending upon whether the process is primarily hemolytic, hypoplastic, or the result of infiltrative disease.[22]

The indications for institution of cytotoxic chemotherapy for macroglobulinemia are quite different from those for multiple myeloma. Macroglobulinemia is generally not a very virulent disease and is compatible with long survival; therefore, *only the symptomatic patient with macroglobulinemia is treated, and then quite cautiously.* In this disease with a relatively benign course, drug-induced marrow aplasia is unacceptable.

ILLUSTRATIVE CASE HISTORY: MACROGLOBULINEMIA

This patient's course is summarized in Figure 13–4. In 1949 the patient, then age 48, noted the onset of menorrhagia and had episodes of epistaxis, and she underwent a hysterectomy. Epistaxis became more frequent and severe over the subsequent years. In 1959 the patient was evaluated for

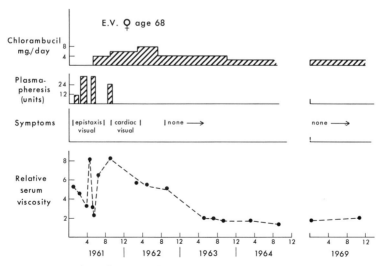

Figure 13–4   Clinical course of a patient with Waldenström's macroglobulinemia who responded to chlorambucil therapy. See case history.

anemia at the University of California Hospitals, San Francisco. She was
found to have an abnormally high serum protein concentration; serum electrophoresis showed a sharp peak in the gamma globulin region (Fig. 13-5).
The abnormal protein migrated as a macroglobulin in the ultracentrifuge. On
the basis of these findings, as well as peripheral blood lymphocytosis and
bone marrow containing "plasmacytoid cells," a diagnosis of Waldenström's
macroglobulinemia was made. No treatment was given other than iron (oral
administration).

In *January 1961*, at age 60, the patient complained of severe epistaxis

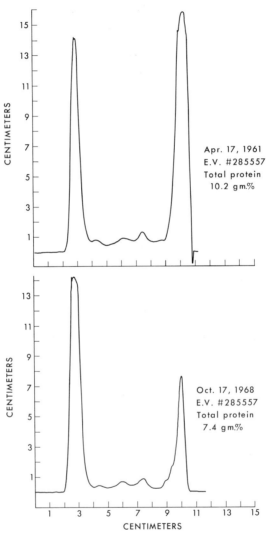

Figure 13–5 Sequential electrophoresis of the serum of the same patient with
Waldenström's macroglobulinemia showed a decrease in the magnitude of the macroglobulin "spike" after chlorambucil therapy.

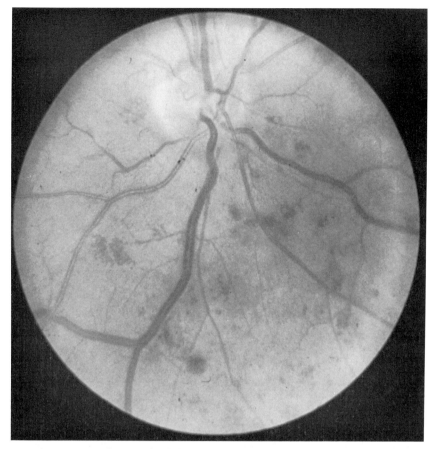

Figure 13-6 Photograph of the retina of the same patient with Waldenström's macroglobulinemia and hyperviscosity syndrome before therapy.

and decreased visual acuity. The relative serum viscosity was 5.1 (normal, 1.8 to 2.0), and funduscopic findings included retinal vein distention and hemorrhages (Fig. 13-6). Ten units of plasma were removed by plasmapheresis, which reduced the serum viscosity to 4.5. Because there was little change in symptoms, an additional 36 units was removed by plasmapheresis over a 30-day period. By this maneuver the serum viscosity was reduced to 3.3, and symptoms were alleviated. Within 2 weeks, however, epistaxis and visual symptoms recurred, and the serum viscosity was found to be 8.1 (*April 11, 1961*). An intensive course of plasmapheresis was started and chlorambucil treatment was begun at an initial dosage of 4 mg. per day.

Over the next 3 months, from May to August 1961, the viscosity gradually rose to 8.3 and the patient began to complain of exertional dyspnea and chest pain as well as visual impairment. Twenty-four units of plasma were removed and the chlorambucil dosage was increased to 6 mg. per day and then to 8 mg. per day. Over the subsequent period of 20 months serum viscosity gradually fell to the normal range and symptoms disappeared. The chlorambucil dosage was adjusted to keep the peripheral white blood count at about 3000 per cu. mm.

As of *December 1969*, when the patient was age 69, 20 years had elapsed since her initial symptoms appeared. She was asymptomatic on a small dose of chlorambucil; the serum viscosity was normal, although an abnormal "spike" was still present in the serum electrophoresis (Fig. 13–2).

COMMENT. This patient is an example of the long natural history of Waldenström's macroglobulinemia possible with judicious therapy. The initial symptoms, related to hyperviscosity (epistaxis and visual disturbances), were briefly controlled by plasmapheresis. However, the paraprotein concentration increased rapidly when plasmapheresis was stopped. The high level of the macroglobulin fell slowly with chlorambucil therapy. Plasmapheresis was reserved for acute symptoms of hyperviscosity.

References

1. Carbone, P. P., Kellerhouse, L. E., and Gehan, E. A.: Plasmacytic myeloma. Amer. J. Med., *42*:937, 1967.
2. Bergsagel, D. E., and Pruzanski, W.: Recognizing and treating plasma cell neoplasia. Postgrad. Med., *43*:200, 1968.
3. Cohn, M.: Natural history of the myeloma. Cold Spr. Harb. Symp. Quant. Biol., *32*:211, 1967.
4. Alexanian, R., Bergsagel, D. E., Migliore, P. J., Vaughn, W. K., and Howe, C. D.: Melphalan therapy for plasma cell myeloma. Blood, *31*:1–10, 1968.
5. Fahey, J. L.: Evidence for heterogeneity of plasma cells: Studies of proteins produced by plasma cell tumors in inbred mice. Ann. New York Acad. Sci., *101*:221, 1962.
6. Finkel, H. E., Yount, W. J., Salmon, S. E., and Schilling, A.: Current concepts in the therapy of multiple myeloma. Med. Clin. N. Amer., *50*:1569–1578, 1966.
7. Waldenström, J.: Melphalan therapy in myelomatosis. Brit. Med. J., *1*:859, 1964.
8. Bergsagel, D. E., Migliore, P. J., and Griffith, K. M.: Myeloma proteins and the clinical response to melphalan therapy. Science, *148*:376, 1965.
9. Korst, D. R., Clifford, G. O., Fowler, W. M., Louis, J., Will, J., and Wilson, H. E.: Multiple myeloma. II. Analysis of cyclophosphamide therapy in 165 patients. J.A.M.A., *189*:156, 1964.
10. Edwards, G. A., and Zawadzki, Z. A.: Extraosseous lesions in plasma cell myeloma, Amer. J. Med., *43*:194, 1967.
11. Bryan, C. W., and Healy, J. K.: Acute renal failure in multiple myeloma. Amer. J. Med., *44*:128, 1968.
12. Anderson, J., and Osgood, E. E.: Acute plasmacytic leukemia responsive to cyclophosphamide. J.A.M.A., *193*:844, 1965.
13. Cohen, P., and Gardner, F. H.: Induction of subacute skeletal fluorosis in a case of multiple myeloma. New Eng. J. Med., *271*:1129, 1964.
14. Lazor, M. Z., and Rosenberg, L. E.: Mechanism of adrenal-steroid reversal of hypercalcemia in multiple myeloma. New Eng. J. Med., *270*:749, 1964.
15. Goldsmith, R. S., and Ingbar, S. H.: Inorganic phosphate treatment of hypercalcemia of diverse etiologies. New Eng. J. Med., *274*:1, 1966.
16. Cline, M. J., and Berlin, N. I.: Studies of the anemia of multiple myeloma. Amer. J. Med., *33*:510, 1962.
17. Salmon, S. E., Samal, B. A., Hayes, D. M., Hosley, H., Miller, S. P., and Schilling, A.: Role of gamma globulin for immunoprophylaxis in multiple myeloma. New Eng. J. Med., *277*:1336, 1967.

17a. Salmon, S. E., and Smith, B. A.: Immunoglobulin synthesis and total body tumor cell number in IgG multiple myeloma. J. Clin. Invest., 49:1114–1121, 1970.
18. McCallister, B. D., Bayrd, E. D., Harrison, E. G., and McGuckin, W. F.: Primary macroglobulinemia. Review with a report on 31 cases and notes on the value of continuous chlorambucil therapy. Amer. J. Med., 43:394, 1967.
19. Macroglobulinemia. Medical Staff Conference. California Med., 108:136, 1968.
20. Solomon, A., and Fahey, J. L.: Plasmapheresis therapy in macroglobulinemia. Ann. Intern. Med., 58:789–800, 1963.
21. Bouroncle, B. A., Datta, P., and Frajola, W. J.: Waldenström's macroglobulinemia: Report of three patients treated with cyclophosphamide. J.A.M.A., 189:729, 1964.
22. Cline, M. J., Solomon, A., Berlin, N. I., and Fahey, J. L.: Anemia in macroglobulinemia. Amer. J. Med., 34:213, 1963.

Additional Recent Bibliography Not Cited in Text

23. Hoogstraten, B., Costa, J., Cuttner, J., Forcier, R. J., Leone, L. A., Harley, J. B., and Glidewell, O. J.: Intermittent melphalan therapy in multiple myeloma. J.A.M.A., 209:251–253, 1969.
24. McArthur, J. R., Athens, J. W., Wintrobe, M. M., and Cartwright, G. E.: Melphalan and myeloma. Experience with a low-dose continuous regimen. Ann. Intern. Med., 72:665–670, 1970.
25. Pruzanski, W., Platts, M. E., and Ogryzlo, M. A.: Leukemic form of immunocytic dyscrasia (plasma cell leukemia). Amer. J. Med., 47:60–74, 1969.
26. MacKenzie, M. R., Fudenberg, H. H., and O'Reilly, R. A.: The hyperviscosity syndrome. I. In IgG myeloma. The role of protein concentration and molecular shape. J. Clin. Invest., 49:15–20, 1970.
27. Fishkin, B. G., Glassy, F. J., Hattersley, P. G., Hirose, F. M., and Spiegelberg, H. L.: IgD multiple myeloma: A report of five cases. Amer. J. Clin. Path., 53:209–214, 1970.

CHAPTER 14

THE CHEMOTHERAPEUTIC TREATMENT OF COMPLICATIONS ASSOCIATED WITH MALIGNANT DISEASE

MALIGNANT PLEURAL EFFUSIONS

Intractable pleural effusions are a frequent and difficult problem in the therapy of the patient with neoplastic disease. Effusions may arise from invasion of the pleura or obstruction of the lymphatic drainage of intrathoracic organs by tumors of epithelial, mesenchymal, or lymphoid origin. This problem is encountered most commonly in carcinoma of the lung, breast, and ovary and in malignant lymphoma.

Numerous therapeutic procedures have been devised, including surgical drainage and obliteration of the pleural space and administration of radioactive agents and cytotoxic drugs and drugs that cause inflammatory reactions with subsequent fibrosis. There is no uniformity of opinion regarding the treatment of choice of intractable pleural effusions. Each treatment center has its own favorite procedure, and no wholly satisfactory comparative study exists in the English literature.

Critical to the evaluation of the claims for any new procedures that involve thoracocentesis and instillation of an agent is the observation that thorough drainage alone will control pleural effusions in a high percentage of cases.[1] If the pleural surfaces infiltrated by tumor can be maintained in apposition for a reasonable period of time, they will frequently adhere and obliterate the pleural space.

The sequential treatment of malignant pleural effusions used at the University of California Hospitals, San Francisco, is outlined in Table 14-1 (refs. 1 to 4). The first approach is to control the malignant

182

process by systemic therapy. Unfortunately this goal is not always attainable, either because the tumor is unresponsive or because bone marrow depression precludes vigorous chemotherapy. In occasional patients, vigorous treatment with an effective diuretic (e.g., chlorothiazide, mercuhydrin, or furosemide) will control effusions or delay reaccumulation. Such diuretic therapy is only a stopgap measure, and is rarely more than temporarily effective. Therefore, in general, attention must be directed specifically toward the neoplastic disease in the pleural space.

When systemic chemotherapy and diuretic agents have failed or are inappropriate, a good practice is to try thoracocentesis twice or even three times to control symptoms, assess the rate of fluid reaccumulation, and, if possible, obliterate the pleural space. If this third maneuver fails to prevent the recurrence of effusion, closed-chest drainage can be established, which, continued for 4 or 5 days, will allow apposition of the pleural surfaces and fibrosis. This procedure can be expected to be successful in about half the patients.

It is frequently more convenient to try nitrogen mustard before instituting closed-chest drainage. The choice is influenced by the clinical situation, the facilities available, and the experience of the physician. Nitrogen mustard may be given in full therapeutic doses up to 0.4 mg. per kg. It is important to realize, however, that this drug is frequently absorbed from the pleural space to exert a systemic effect. Therefore, the dosage should be reduced in cases of bone marrow depression. It is important to remove as much fluid as possible before giving the nitrogen mustard.

It is rarely necessary to use quinacrine to control effusions. The previously described therapeutic techniques usually suffice. When quinacrine is used in otherwise resistant effusions, it is usually effective but at the cost of considerable discomfort to the patient, local pain, and high fever. The drug appears to act by setting up an inflammatory reaction within the pleural space followed by fibrosis.

Another possible therapeutic approach to the control of effusions is the use of β-emitting radioisotopes, which locally irradiate the

TABLE 14-1 *Suggested Sequential Treatment of Malignant Pleural Effusions*

	REFERENCE
1. Control of the malignant process by systemic therapy	
2. Diuretic agents	
3. Thoracocentesis (x 2 or x 3)	
4. Closed chest drainage	1
5. Nitrogen mustard (intrapleural)	2
6. Quinacrine	3
7. Radioisotopes	4

pleural space. Both radioactive gold and radioactive phosphorus have been used. We have tended to avoid the use of radioisotopes because of the cost (gold), the dangers of systemic irradiation and bone marrow depression, and the difficulty of using therapeutic doses of radioisotopes when patients are in an open ward.

Other agents and techniques have been used to control effusions, including new drugs, e.g., 5-fluorouracil,[5] and surgical decortication of the lung. It is too early to judge the effectiveness of drugs other than alkylating agents, and in my opinion surgical decortication is like taking a sledge hammer to kill a fly.

SPINAL CORD COMPRESSION

The symptoms of spinal cord compression constitute an emergency. Treatment must be prompt, and optimal treatment requires a smoothly functioning, multidisciplinary team. We have found no substitute for close and frequent communication among the physicians involved in the care of the patient with spinal cord compression.

A fairly extensive review of the treatment of spinal cord compression from metastatic carcinoma (including lymphoma) has appeared recently.[6]

The policy at the University of California Hospitals, San Francisco, has been to place the patient with spinal cord compression in one of two categories: slowly evolving compression (days to weeks), or rapidly evolving compression (hours to days). Obviously the patient must be observed around the clock to make certain that his disease does not progress from the first to the second category. If the patient has slowly progressive disease, our policy has been to obtain a myelogram. A neurosurgeon is always in attendance in the event that a partial block is converted into a complete block and emergency laminectomy is required. Once the level of the lesion has been ascertained, nitrogen mustard is given in a dose sufficient to induce remission (cf. Table 12-4) and x-ray therapy is begun immediately, directed to the involved site and several vertebral spaces above and below it. It can be argued that Thiotepa should be given rather than nitrogen mustard, since Thiotepa is less likely to provoke vomiting.

If the patient is in the second category and has signs of rapidly progressive compression, or if the course of compression is uncertain, laminectomy should be performed, followed within hours by radiation therapy and chemotherapy. Loss of cord function by lymphomatous compression is rarely reversible; therefore, it is best to operate if there is any doubt about the rate of progression or the response to other treatment.

ILLUSTRATIVE CASE HISTORY: RECURRENT MALIG-
NANT PLEURAL EFFUSIONS

The clinical course and response to therapy are illustrated in Figures
14–1 to 14–4.

The patient had been well until *September 1968* (age 59 years), when a
left radical mastectomy was performed for infiltrating ductal carcinoma.
Because 1 of every 20 lymph nodes examined was positive for carcinoma,
the left axillary area was irradiated postoperatively (total dose, 5000 rads).
In *February 1969*, the patient returned to the hospital for an elective chole-
cystectomy. At that time a hard nodule 2 cm. in length was discovered on the
left chest wall just outside the field of the previous irradiation. The diagnosis
at biopsy of this nodule was carcinoma, and the patient was given another
course of irradiation (total dose, 5300 rads).

The following month (*March 1969*) the patient complained of dyspnea.
Fluid aspirated from the left pleural space contained malignant cells. Pleural
effusions recurred at 2- to 3-week intervals in amounts sufficient to produce
symptoms, and repeated thoracenteses were performed for relief.

In *May 1969*, the patient was started on a regimen of estrogen, given
orally. During estrogen therapy, skin metastases, which had first appeared
in April 1969, increased in size; also there was no diminution in the rate of
accumulation of pleural effusions. Estrogen was discontinued, and over the
next 14 weeks the patient was given brief trials with testosterone and then
with 5-FU. Both agents were ineffective.

In *October 1969*, thoracentesis was performed and Thiotepa (30 mg.)
was instilled in the left pleural space. This procedure was well tolerated, and
the rate of accumulation of fluid obviously diminished over the subsequent 6
weeks. However, in late *November 1969*, symptoms of pleural effusion recurred, including exertional dyspnea.

After removal of 2000 ml. of serosanguineous fluid from the left chest, 10
mg. of nitrogen mustard was instilled intrapleurally. The patient was moved

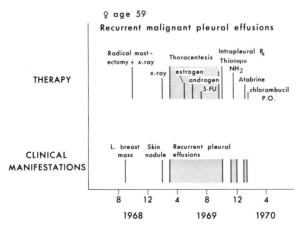

Figure 14–1   Clinical course and response to therapy of a patient with malignant
pleural effusions resulting from carcinoma of the breast. See case history.

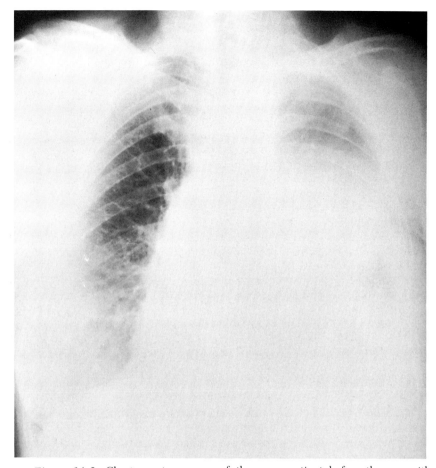

Figure 14-2   Chest roentgenogram of the same patient before therapy with intrapleural Atabrine.

about in various positions to promote distribution of the alkylating agent. She tolerated the procedure well except for a 24-hour period of nausea and repeated emesis. A chest roentgenogram taken after thoracentesis showed a marked decrease in the amount of pleural effusion; only a small amount of residual fluid was present at the left base. However, physical examination 2 days later disclosed reaccumulation of pleural fluid on the left side; again serosanguineous fluid (1800 ml.) was removed.

Chest roentgenograms revealed no further accumulation of fluid during the following month. However, early in *January 1970*, the patient returned to the hospital with recurrence of her previous symptoms and enlargement of skin nodules. An Intracath was inserted in the left pleural space under fluoroscopic guidance and was taped in place before the instillation of Atabrine, 200 mg. in 25 ml. of normal saline. The chest tube was drained under closed water-seal for 2 days. The patient's temperature rose to 39° C., and she experienced mild nausea and pleuritic chest pain as a result of the

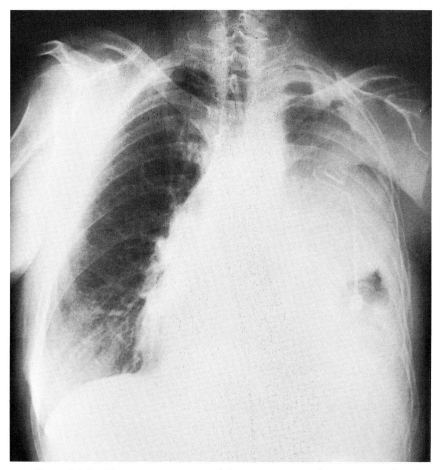

Figure 14–3 Chest roentgenogram of the same patient after insertion of a tube for drainage and instillation of Atabrine.

Atabrine therapy. She recovered sufficiently to be discharged from the hospital 4 days later. At this time oral administration of chlorambucil for systemic disease was started. At a follow-up examination 6 weeks later, there was minimal pleural effusion and an early response of the metastatic skin nodules to the chlorambucil therapy was apparent.

COMMENT: A series of progressively more vigorous attacks on recurrent pleural effusions in this patient with metastatic carcinoma of the breast finally resulted in control of the effusions after about 1 year. The sequential therapy consisted of repeated thoracenteses and intrapleural administration of Thiotepa, nitrogen mustard, and Atabrine. During the attack on the pleural effusions, trials with hormonal and chemotherapeutic agents were unsuccessful in controlling the systemic disease.

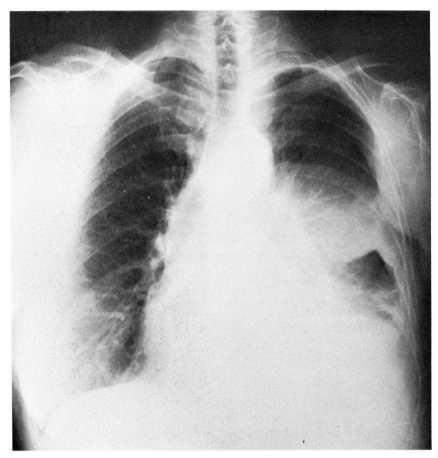

Figure 14–4 Chest roentgenogram of the same patient 4 weeks after instillation of Atabrine.

REFERENCES

1. Lambert, C. J., Shah, H. H., Urschel, H. C., Jr., and Paulson, D. L.: Treatment of malignant pleural effusions by closed trocar tube drainage. Ann. Thorac. Surg., 3:1–5, 1967.
2. Weisberger, A. S., Levine, B., and Storaasli, J. P.: The use of nitrogen mustard in the treatment of serous effusions of neoplastic origin. J.A.M.A., 159:1704, 1955.
3. Dollinger, M. R., Krakoff, I. H., and Karnofsky, D. A.: Quinacrine (Atabrine) in the treatment of neoplastic effusions. Ann. Intern. Med., 66:249, 1967.
4. Kent, E. M., and Moses, C.: Radioactive isotopes in palliative management of carcinomatosis of the pleura. J. Thorac. Surg., 22:503, 1951.
5. Suhrland, L. G., and Weisberger, A. S.: Intracavitary 5-fluorouracil in malignant effusions. Arch. Intern. Med., 116:431, 1965.
6. Silverberg, I. J.: Management of effusions. Oncology, 24:26, 1970.
7. Millburn, L., Hibbs, G. G., and Hendrickson, F. R.: Treatment of spinal cord compression from metastatic carcinoma. Cancer, 21:447, 1968.

CHAPTER 15

PROSPECTS FOR THE FUTURE

It is probable that the future advances in the chemotherapeutic management of cancer will occur in three main areas: the discovery and exploitation of new drugs, the more effective use of well-established agents, and the development of facilities for intensive supportive care of the cancer patient.

NEW DRUGS

The discovery of effective new anticancer drugs in the past few years has been impressive. The number of potentially useful drugs exceeds our capacity to do rigorous phase I testing in man. Many of the new compounds resemble traditional agents in their mode of antitumor action but differ in their pharmacologic characteristics. For example, daunomycin is an antibiotic, which, like actinomycin-D, binds to certain base residues of DNA.[1, 2] Unlike actinomycin, however, daunomycin appears to be effective in childhood leukemia. BCNU acts like an alkylating agent, but unlike the standard alkylating agents BCNU now appears to be effective in treating brain tumors, e.g., glioblastoma, perhaps because of its lipid solubility.[3]

Other new agents represent a totally new mode of attack on malignant cells. One is L-asparaginase, which, by destroying the amino acid L-asparagine, exploits the fact that certain tumors require exogenous L-asparagine, whereas most normal tissues do not.[4, 5] The discovery of this enzyme in guinea pig serum[6] and its subsequent isolation from mutant strains of *Escherichia coli*[5] have provided a new impetus to cancer chemotherapy. Although L-asparaginase itself is only moderately effective against certain human leukemias and lymphomas, the exploitation of a qualitative difference between normal and neoplastic cells has led to a new phase of endeavor. Undoubtedly other modes of exploiting the difference in asparagine metabolism in normal and neoplastic tissues will be discovered (for example, the use of asparagine analogs). It is to be hoped that other differences between normal and neoplastic tissues will also be discovered.

Another mode of attacking the cancer cell may involve the use of pharmacologic amounts of certain metabolites normally found in trace quantities. The results obtained with such compounds in animal tumor model systems have been truly remarkable.[7]

Drug Screening

How does the biologist know when he has a potentially useful anticancer drug? Phrased another way, how reliable are our present animal tumor models for predicting a clinically useful drug? How good are our drug screening programs? The answer seems to be that the animal model systems, although good, are not perfect. For example, our current screening systems would select most but not all of the presently useful drugs.[8] Improved and more economic drug-screening programs are critical to the identification of new chemotherapeutic agents. It should be acknowledged that to date the national screening program under the aegis of the National Institutes of Health has done a superb job in screening new anticancer drugs.

Pharmacologic studies of new drugs in man are often slow and always extremely difficult. Consequently, it is probable that some potentially useful agents are put aside as the result of poorly performed or inadequate phase I testing in man. We are just beginning to learn how to do proper phase I studies,[9] and it is likely that we can anticipate a more rapid rate of evaluating new drugs in the future.

In Table 15-1 (references 1 to 6, 9 to 15) is a partial list of the

TABLE 15-1 *New Drugs Under Study at the Cancer Research Institute, University of California, San Francisco*

AGENT	TUMORS TREATED	REFERENCE
L-asparaginase	Acute leukemia, lymphomas	4–6
BCNU (1, 3 bis-(β-chloroethyl)-1-nitrosourea)	Brain tumors, lymphomas, melanoma	3
Daunomycin	Acute leukemia and solid tumors of childhood	1, 2
Dibromomannitol	Various	9
Hexamethylmelamine	Bronchogenic carcinoma	10
Mithromycin	Various	11, 12
Streptonigrin	Various	13
Streptozotocin	Various	14
Thioguanine (in combination with cytosine arabinoside)	Acute leukemia	15

new drugs under study at the Cancer Research Institute of the University of California, San Francisco. Considering the number of cancer centers in the United States, it becomes obvious that the new anticancer drugs being studied in man are numbered in the hundreds.

MORE EFFECTIVE USE OF ESTABLISHED AGENTS

The difficulties of pharmacologic studies in man apply to well-known agents as well as new drugs. Only one example of this phenomenon need be cited. For many years methotrexate was administered orally in low doses. Under these conditions the drug was rarely effective for inducing remissions in acute lymphocytic leukemia, but was an effective "maintaining" agent when remission had been induced by other drugs. With review of the pharmacology of methotrexate and re-examination of the data from animal tumor model systems, the format of its administration was changed and the drug was given parenterally in short intensive courses.[16] Under these conditions methotrexate is an effective inducing agent.

It appears likely that the more effective use of established drugs will come from the following: animal model systems to test dosage schedules and pharmacologic characteristics; combinations of drugs with differing modes of action; pharmacokinetic studies; the use of drugs in a manner that maximizes their effectiveness during the cycle of cell replication; and in vitro test systems for determining the efficacy of a given drug against a tumor.

Animal Models

The use of animal tumor model systems to determine optimal schedules of drug administration has resulted in several successful clinical trials. Such model systems have demonstrated that short courses of intensive therapy with certain drugs are superior to low-dose, prolonged treatment.

The limitations of the animal tumor model in determining drug treatment in man are many, however. The most obvious are the species-dependent differences in drug metabolism and response to tumor and the differences in kinetics of spontaneous tumor growth in man and animals.

Combination Therapy

Although the use of combinations of drugs is standard practice at many cancer research centers, such therapy cannot be considered "standard" for the general medical community.

The combination of multiple agents has already produced striking results in patients with stage IV Hodgkin's disease[17, 18] (see Chap. 12) and acute lymphocytic leukemia[19] (see Chap. 10). There is no doubt that the future will produce effective drug combinations for other hematologic malignancies and solid tumors.[20, 21] Combination therapy of solid tumors other than the rare choriocarcinoma, soft tissue sarcomas, and testicular neoplasms has had only limited trial at the present time.

Pharmacokinetic Studies

Pharmacokinetic studies of drugs and their metabolites hold promise of more sophisticated and more rational drug administration schedules that take advantage of information regarding rates of distribution, catabolism, and excretion of drug and the extent of binding to serum proteins and uptake by cells. A few anticancer drugs have been studied by these methods but generally not in depth. The best studies have been concerned with drugs other than chemotherapeutic agents. It is possible that difficulties will be encountered because of the problems in identifying which drug metabolite is the active one (e.g., cyclophosphamide metabolites) and also because of the extremely minute quantities of certain anticancer drugs that are effective (e.g., 10^{-9} M vincristine). These minute quantities make even such sensitive techniques as gas chromatography grossly inadequate.

CELL CYCLE. Many of the commonly used chemotherapeutic agents are cell cycle-specific, that is, effective during a particular phase of the cell cycle.* Pharmacokinetic studies of anticancer drugs and schedules of administration should take into account the kinetics of a population of malignant cells.[22] If a population of malignant cells could be made to divide synchronously, the administration of a given drug could be timed to correspond to that phase of the replicative cycle when the drug is most effective. The major problems are how to induce synchronous division and how to mobilize dormant G0 cells into the replicative cycle. The attempts thus far have involved phasing the cells with one set of agents before giving cytocidal doses of a second set of agents. The preliminary results are encouraging.

In Vitro Tests

In vitro test systems can be used to predict the effect of a given drug on a given tumor in vivo.[23] The clinical microbiologist routinely uses laboratory screening tests to select the appropriate antibiotic for the treatment of a patient with bacterial infection. Can the same

---

*Chapter 1 describes the importance of the cell replication cycle as a determinant of the effectiveness of most useful agents.

principle of interaction of drugs and target cells in vitro be applied for the selection of agents in treating patients with cancer? The answer is a qualified "yes."

Attempts to develop in vitro systems for predicting the in vivo effectiveness of anticancer drugs extend back to the early 1940s. Several experimental models have been devised. If the site of action of a chemotherapeutic agent is known, the effect of the drug on a given enzyme or metabolic pathway in isolated tumor cells can be compared with its clinical effectiveness. If the primary site of action of an agent is unknown, the problem is more difficult. Test systems for such drugs are potentially feasible, provided the drugs exert a secondary effect on cellular metabolism that is measurable and that correlates with clinical effectiveness. Many secondary effects have been examined, including those on oxygen consumption, carbohydrate metabolism, nucleic acid synthesis, and exclusion of supravital stains.

Whether or not the site of action is known, certain minimal conditions must be met: (1) The drug must be active in the form in which it is added to the in vitro system or must be converted to an active form by the constituents of that system. (2) The metabolism of the malignant cells in vivo and in vitro must be sufficiently similar so that drug effects under the two conditions are comparable. (3) There must be sufficient time for drug action to become manifest. (4) Finally, a representative sample of the tumor must be obtained for testing. This last consideration is not generally a problem with the hematologic malignancies, but it is an almost insurmountable obstacle in the case of solid tumors, which are characterized by geographic heterogeneity of cell population and viability. In view of these complex requirements, it is not surprising that in vitro tests in general have been either unreliable or too cumbersome for routine use. It is unfortunate that one of the best correlations between an in vitro test system and the clinical response occurs with a drug that is used only rarely.[24]

The outlook is not entirely gloomy, however. Recently the assiduous application of a long-recognized principle has begun to pay dividends. In the case of all commonly used anticancer agents (except L-asparaginase), the drug must enter a malignant cell before it can exert a cytotoxic effect. If it is exluded or fails to bind to its intracellular target molecules, the drug will be ineffective. With the use of radioactively labeled drugs and representative populations of leukemia cells, this principle has recently been applied with some success to in vitro test systems.[25] It is obvious, however, that although the drug must penetrate a malignant cell, this is not necessarily sufficient for a cytotoxic effect. Therefore, test systems based solely on drug uptake can exclude ineffective agents but cannot always predict effective ones.

At present, one must not ask too much of predictive systems for anticancer drugs. The clinical response to a chemotherapeutic agent depends on many factors in addition to a reduction in the number of neoplastic cells. The bacteriologist asks that his in vitro test answer only two questions. Will the drug kill bacteria? At what concentrations is it effective? Similarly, at best, the chemotherapist can hope to gain information about dose-dependent cytotoxicity against malignant cells. It may be that in vitro test systems for cancer drugs will be most useful in indicating drugs or drug combinations that are least likely to be effective for a given patient. Even this modest goal is desirable.

INTENSIVE SUPPORTIVE THERAPY

At the present time, the leading causes of death in the hematologic malignancies are bleeding and overwhelming infections. These are also major causes of death in patients with solid tumors treated by intensive chemotherapy. Bleeding can usually be ascribed directly to thrombocytopenia resulting from either the underlying neoplastic disease or myelosuppressive chemotherapy. Only rarely do other defects in the hemostatic mechanism contribute to the bleeding diathesis in patients with hematologic malignancies.

Several factors contribute to the susceptibility to infection of this group of patients: reduced numbers of granulocytes, impaired granulocyte function, and defective cellular and humoral immunologic response.

The solutions to the twin problems of bleeding and infection are potentially at hand. In theory, if platelets could be administered to the thrombocytopenic patient with complete freedom, bleeding might be prevented. In practice, this objective is attainable in part by the use of freshly prepared platelets for transfusion. There are two limitations. The first is financial: In an adult with significant thrombocytopenia, one must administer platelet concentrates from 8 to 12 units of blood. In a large urban center, this costs roughly $300 to $500. In view of the fact that such transfusions may have to be repeated at 48- to 72-hour intervals, this form of therapy rapidly becomes prohibitively expensive. With reorganization of blood-banking practices to fractionate each unit of blood into all its component parts, high cost may not be as great a problem in the future.

The selection of antigenically compatible platelets may obviate the problem of the development of platelet antibodies. The use of frozen platelets in the future may also improve the acquisition of large stocks of fresh platelets. It is likely, therefore, that eventually the bleeding problem will be solved.

The restoration of host defense mechanisms against micro-organisms presents a more complex problem. The abnormalities of humoral antibody present in many of the lymphoproliferative diseases can be corrected at least in part by the administration of immunoglobulin concentrates. At present such concentrates are deficient in IgA. Such a deficiency will probably be repaired in the future. The restoration of adequate numbers of functioning granulocytes is a more difficult problem. The studies from the National Cancer Institute have shown that cells from patients with chronic myelocytic leukemia in relapse will probably function to combat sepsis in patients with acute leukemia who have no circulating granulocytes or granulocyte reserves. Such treatment with donated granulocytes has inherent limitations. The most obvious is the rarity of patients with chronic myelocytic leukemia whose disease is in such poor control that they have high levels (greater than 50,000 per cu. mm.) of circulating granulocytes and are therefore suitable leukocyte donors. An attempt has been made by the National Cancer Institute in concert with the IBM Corporation to circumvent this limitation by developing a machine — a white cell separator — that would efficiently and selectively extract leukocytes from normal donors. Unfortunately such machines are more efficient for separating lymphocytes than granulocytes.

It is possible that the answer to the problem of obtaining granulocytes and therapy improving the patient's defense functions may again lie in the reorganization of blood-banking techniques, so that each unit of blood is fractionated to yield its leukocytes as well as other components. Such techniques, combined with improved freezing and storage methodology, could provide a large source of normal and effective phagocytic leukocytes.

Another mode of attacking this problem of infection has been to attempt to protect the patient from microbial flora, both his own and environmental.[26] The initial approach used a combination of antibiotics and a "life island," which encased the patient in a sterile plastic environment. The limitations of the "life island" led to the trial of "laminar flow" rooms, with high-efficiency bacteriologic filters and based on principles derived from the aerospace industry, in which particle-free environments have been critical in certain phases of fabrication and assembly processes. That such protective environments as "life islands" and laminar air flow units will, in fact, effectively protect the patient against infection seems to me, on the basis of existing information, to be doubtful. Therefore, the provision of normal granulocytes will probably be the means of combating the problem of resistant infection in the future.

The recent advances in research will benefit the cancer patient provided the specialized research unit communicates these advances to the practicing physician.

Since cancer chemotherapy is still a relatively new discipline, the "state of the art" is not universally appreciated within the professional medical community. It is already apparent, however, that this gap is being closed.

REFERENCES

1. Kim, J. H., Gelhard, A. S., Djordjevic, B., Kim, S. H., and Perez, A. G.: Action of daunomycin on the nucleic acid metabolism and viability of HeLa cells. Cancer Res., 28:2437–2442, 1968.
2. Tan, C., Tasaka, H., Yu, K.-P., Murphy, M. L., and Karnofsky, D. A.: Daunomycin, an antitumor antibiotic, in the treatment of neoplastic disease. Cancer, 20:333, 1967.
3. Lessner, H. E.: BCNU (1, 3, bis-(β-chloroethyl)-1-nitrosourea)–effects on advanced Hodgkin's disease and other neoplasia. Cancer, 22:451, 1968.
4. Oettgen, H. F., Old, L. J., Boyse, E. A., Campbell, H. A., Philips, F. S., Clarkson, B. D., Tallal, L., Leeper, R. D., Schwartz, M. K., and Kim, J. H.: Inhibition of leukemias in man by L-asparaginase. Cancer Res., 27:2619–2631, 1967.
5. Schein, P. S., Rakieten, N., Gordon, B. M., Davis, R. D., and Rall, D. P.: The toxicity of Escherichia coli L-asparaginase. Cancer Res., 29:426, 1969.
6. Broome, J. D.: Evidence that the L-asparaginase activity of guinea pig serum is responsible for its antilymphoma effects. Nature, 191:1114, 1961.
7. Apple, M. A., and Greenberg, D. M.: Arrest of cancer in mice by therapy with normal metabolites. I. 2-oxopropanal (NSC-79019). Cancer Chemother. Rep., 51:455–464, 1967.
8. Venditti, J. M., and Abbott, B. J.: Studies on oncolytic agents from natural sources. Correlations of activity against animal tumors and clinical effectiveness. Lloydia, 30:332–348, 1967.
9. Casazza, A. R., Cahn, E. L., and Carbone, P. P.: Preliminary studies with dibromomannitol (NSC 94100) in patients with chronic myelogenous leukemia. Cancer Chemother. Rep., 51:91, 1967.
10. Wilson, W. L., Schroeder, J. M., Bisel, H. F., Mrazek, R., and Hummel, R. P.: Phase II study of hexamethylmelamine (NSC 13875). Cancer, 23:132–136, 1969.
11. Brown, J. H., and Kennedy, B. J.: Mithramycin in the treatment of disseminated testicular neoplasms. New Eng. J. Med., 272:111, 1965.
12. Kofman, S., and Eisenstein, R.: Mithramycin in the treatment of disseminated cancer. Cancer Chemother. Rep., 32:77, 1963.
13. Miller, D. S., Laszlo, J., McCarty, K. S., Guild, W. R., and Hochstein, P.: Mechanism of action of streptonigrin in leukemia cells. Cancer Res., 27:632, 1967.
14. Murray-Lyon, I. M., Eddleston, A. L. W. F., Williams, R., Brown, M., Hogbin, B. M., Bennett, A., Edwards, J. C., and Taylor, K. W.: Treatment of multiple-hormone-producing malignant islet-cell carcinoma with streptozotocin. Lancet, 2:895–898, 1968.
15. Gee, T. S., Yu, K. P., Augustin, B. T., Krakoff, I. H., and Clarkson, B. D.: Combination therapy of adult acute leukemia with thioguanine (TG) and 1-B-D-arabino-furanosylcytosine (CA) (abstract). Proc. Amer. Assoc. Cancer Res., 9:23, 1968.
16. Djerassi, I., Farber, S., Abir, E., and Neikirk, W.: Continuous infusion of methotrexate in children with acute leukemia. Cancer, 20:233, 1967.
17. Zubrod, C. G.: New developments in the chemotherapy of the leukemias and lymphomas. In Plenary Session Papers, XII Congress, International Society of Hematology, New York, 1968, page 32.
18. Moxley, J. H., III, De Vita, V. T., Brace, K., and Frei, E., III: Intensive combination chemotherapy and x-irradiation in Hodgkin's disease. Cancer Res., 27:1258–1263, 1967.
19. Henderson, E. S.: Combination chemotherapy of acute lymphocytic leukemia of childhood. Cancer Res., 27:2570, 1967.
20. Nathanson, L., Hall, T. C., Schilling, A., and Miller, S.: Concurrent combination chemotherapy of solid tumors: Experience with a three-drug regimen and review of the literature. Cancer Res., 29:419, 1969.

21. Goldin, A., Venditti, J. M., Mantel, N., Kline, I., and Gang, M.: Evaluation of combination chemotherapy with three drugs. Cancer Res., 28:950–960, 1968.
22. Rall, D. P.: Selective aspects of chemotherapy in acute leukemia and Burkitt's tumor. Cancer, 21:575–579, 1968.
23. Cline, M. J., and Rosenbaum, E.: Prediction of *in vivo* cytotoxicity of chemotherapeutic agents by their *in vitro* effect on leukocytes from patients with acute leukemia. Cancer Res., 28:2516–2521, 1968.
24. Fallon, H. J., Frei, E., III, and Freireich, E. J.: Correlations of the biochemical and clinical effects of 6-azauridine in patients with leukemia. Amer. J. Med., 33:526, 1962.
25. Kessel, D., Hall, T. C., and Roberts, D.: Modes of uptake of methotrexate by normal and leukemic human leukocytes *in vitro* and their relation to drug response. Cancer Res., 28:564–570, 1968.
26. Bodey, G. P., Hart, J., Freireich, E. J., and Frei, E., III: Studies of a patient isolator unit and prophylactic antibiotics in cancer chemotherapy. General techniques and preliminary results. Cancer, 22:1018–1026, 1968.

Additional Recent Bibliography Not Cited in Text

27. Skipper, H. E.: Improvement of the model systems. Cancer Res., 29:2329–2333, 1969.
28. Schabel, F. M., Jr.: The use of tumor growth kinetics in planning "curative" chemotherapy of advanced solid tumors. Cancer Res., 29:2384–2389, 1969.
29. Perry, S.: Reduction of toxicity in cancer chemotherapy. Cancer Res., 29:2319–2325, 1969.
30. Bodey, G. P., Freireich, E. J., and Frei, E., III: Studies of patients in a laminar air flow unit. Cancer, 24:972–980, 1969.

INDEX

Page numbers in *italics* refer to illustrations; (t) refers to tables.

199